T0385715

Iranian Love Stories

Iranian Love Stories

I can assure you, this country is a paradise for women. I'm a queen here.

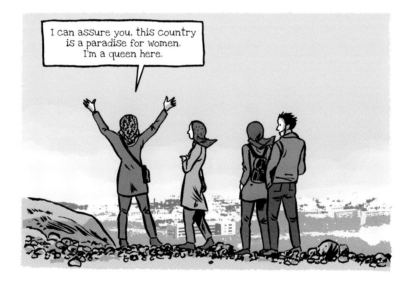

SCRIPT

JANE DEUXARD

ART

DELOUPY

graphic mundi

Do these young Iranians still dream of a regime change?

Jane Deuxard gained their trust. They are all in their twenties and agreed to talk about politics, in spite of the risks. What concerns them more are their love stories, as fraught as they are.

How can you meet someone in a society that forbids it? How do you flirt? How do you choose a husband or a wife? In spite of traditional customs and the current regime...

Jane Deuxard worked covertly. Journalists are not welcome in Iran.

The recent nuclear accord and a president who is considered a reformer may suggest that the regime is easing. But "it isn't so," according to Jamileh, Soban, Vahid, Saeedeh...

Rare testimonies, from across the country. A portrait of Iranian youth. Voices we never hear.

Foreign journalists are not welcome in Iran.
And even less so ever since the demonstrations following President Mahmoud Ahmadinejad's reelection in 2009.

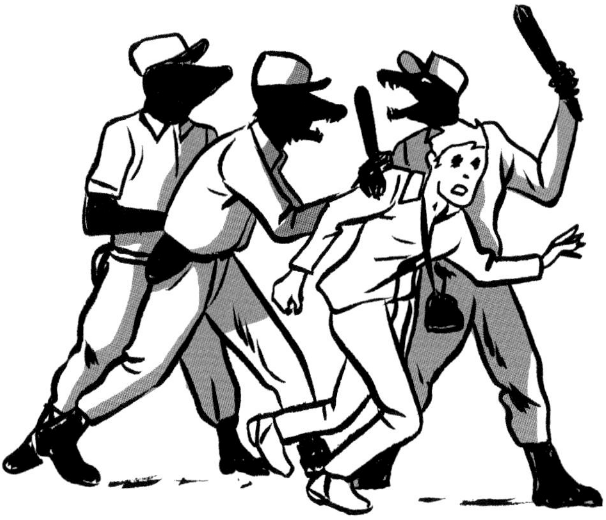

We went covertly.

We are a couple, both journalists, but we're not married. You need to be married to get a hotel room.

Two rings did the trick.

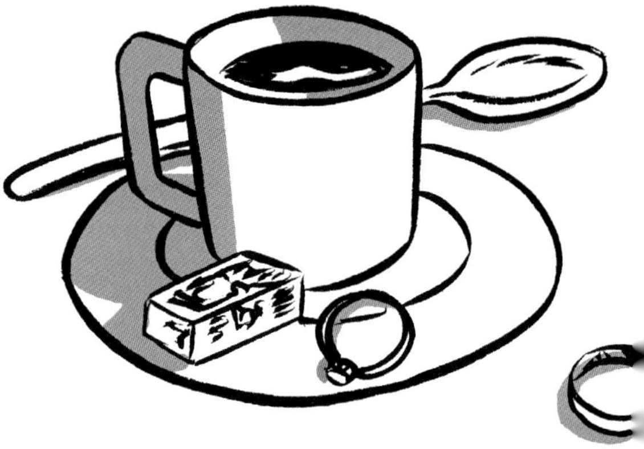

Women must wear a veil in public.
Even in the car and hotel lobbies.
The veil and a three-quarter-length coat.

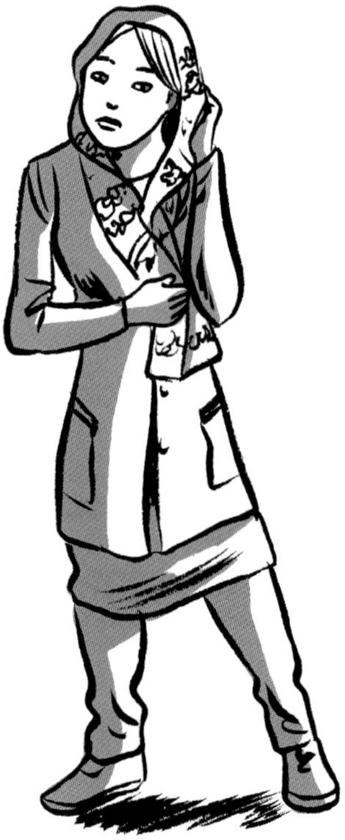

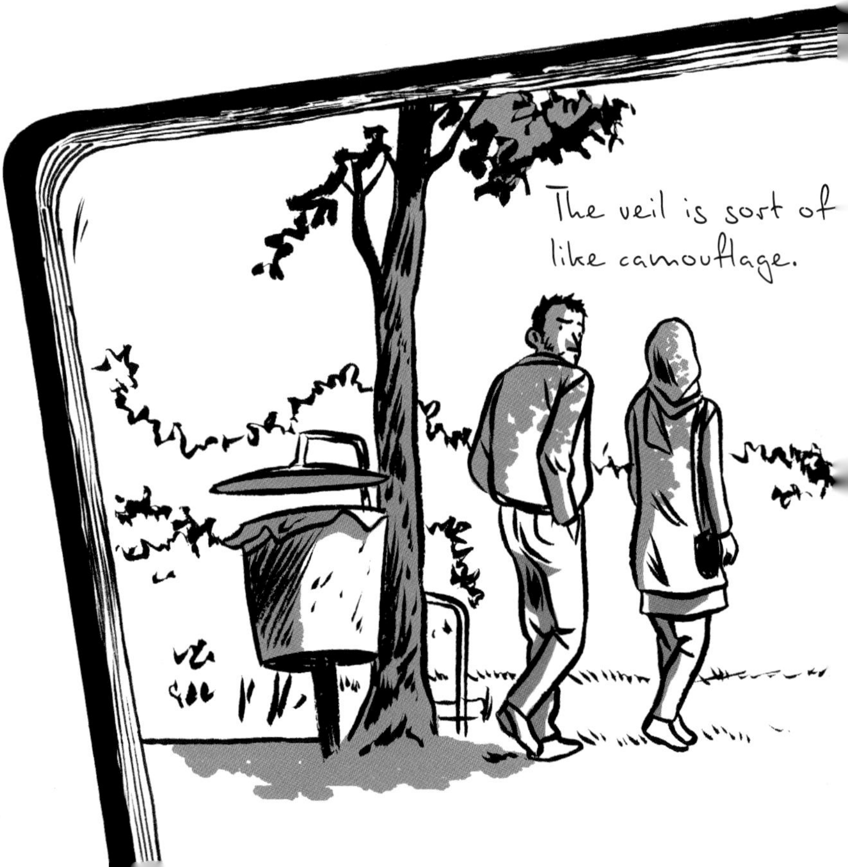
The veil is sort of like camouflage.

GILA, 26,
downtown Tehran.

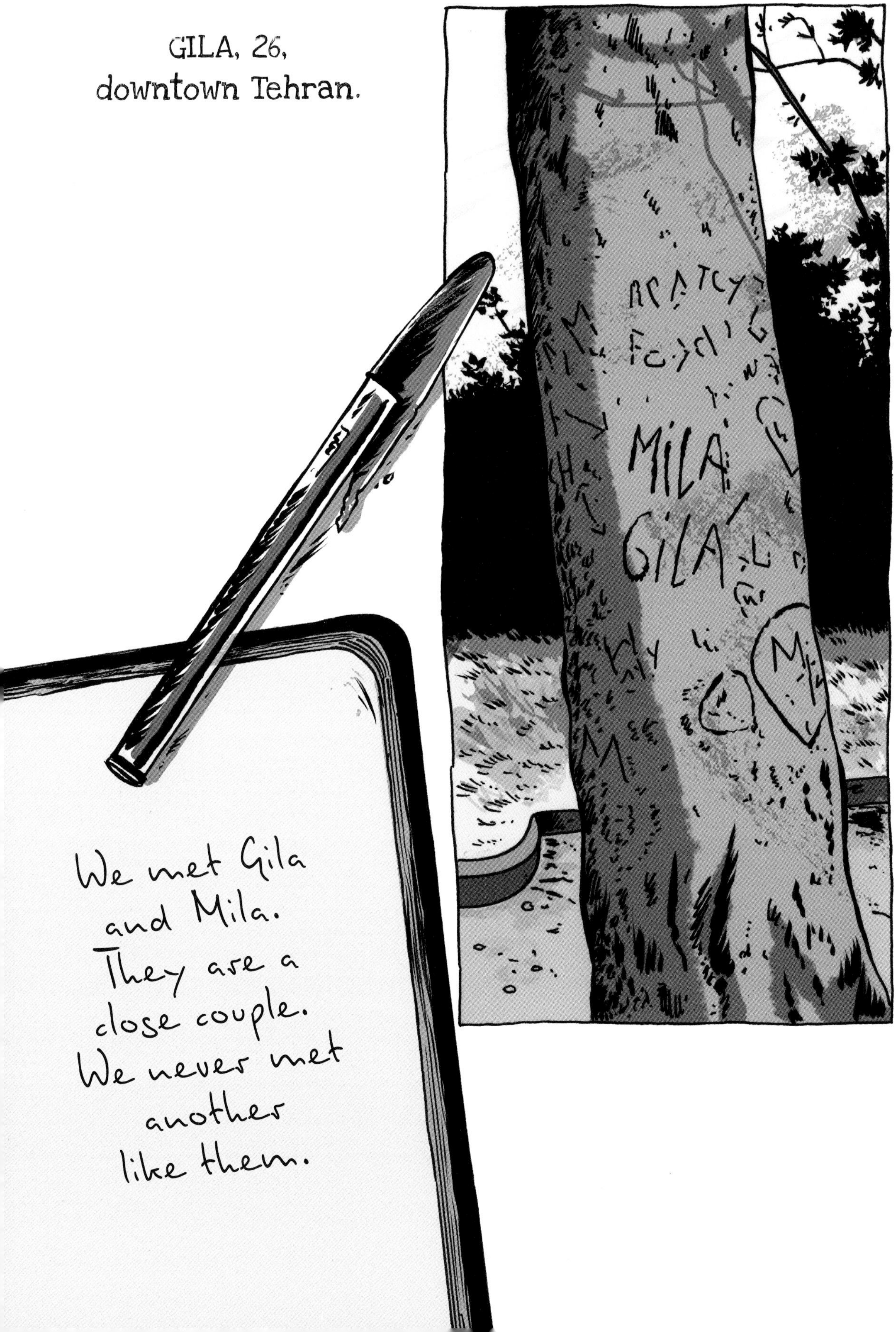
MILA
GILA
We met Gila and Mila. They are a close couple. We never met another like them.

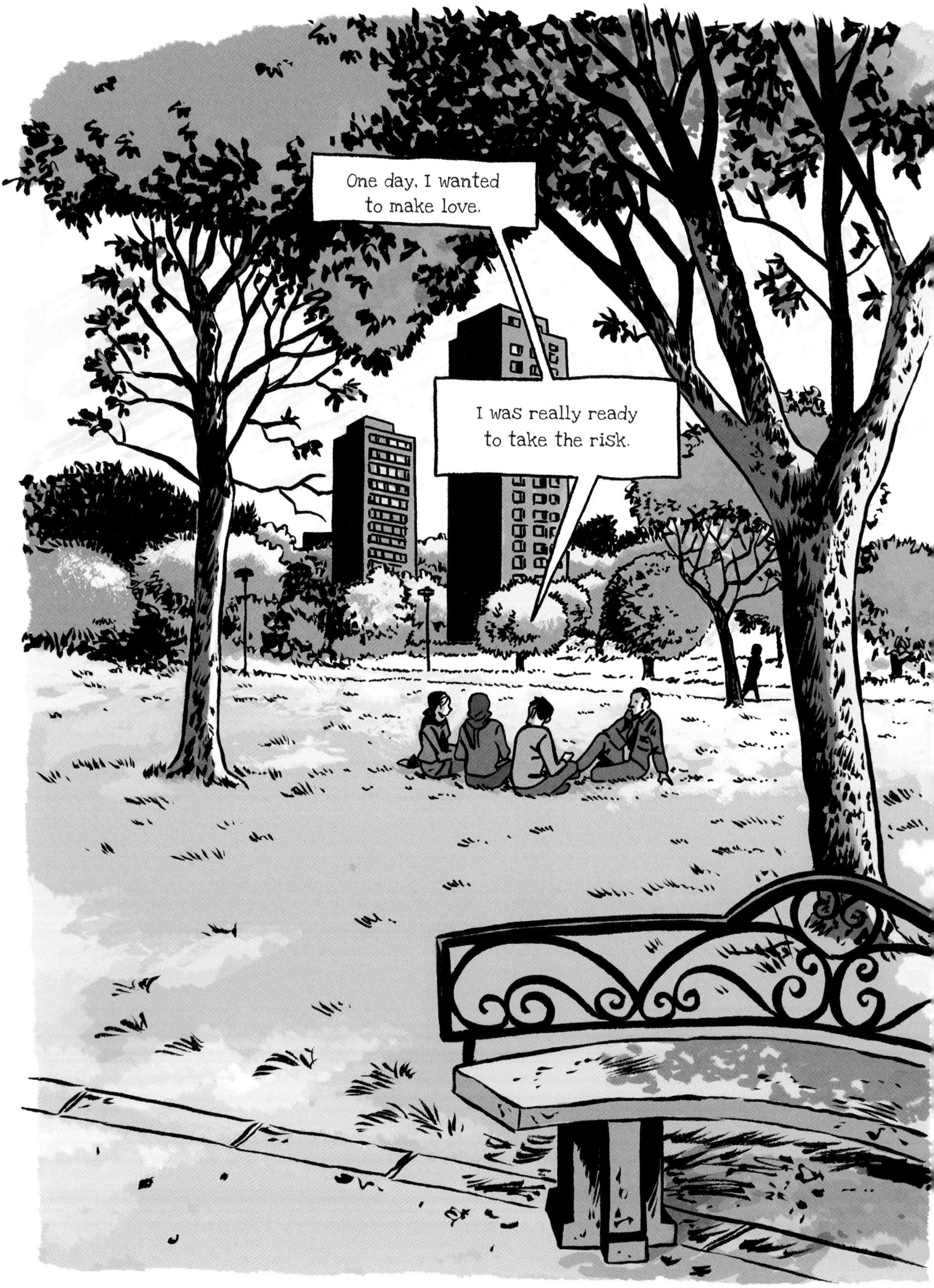
One day, I wanted to make love.
I was really ready to take the risk.

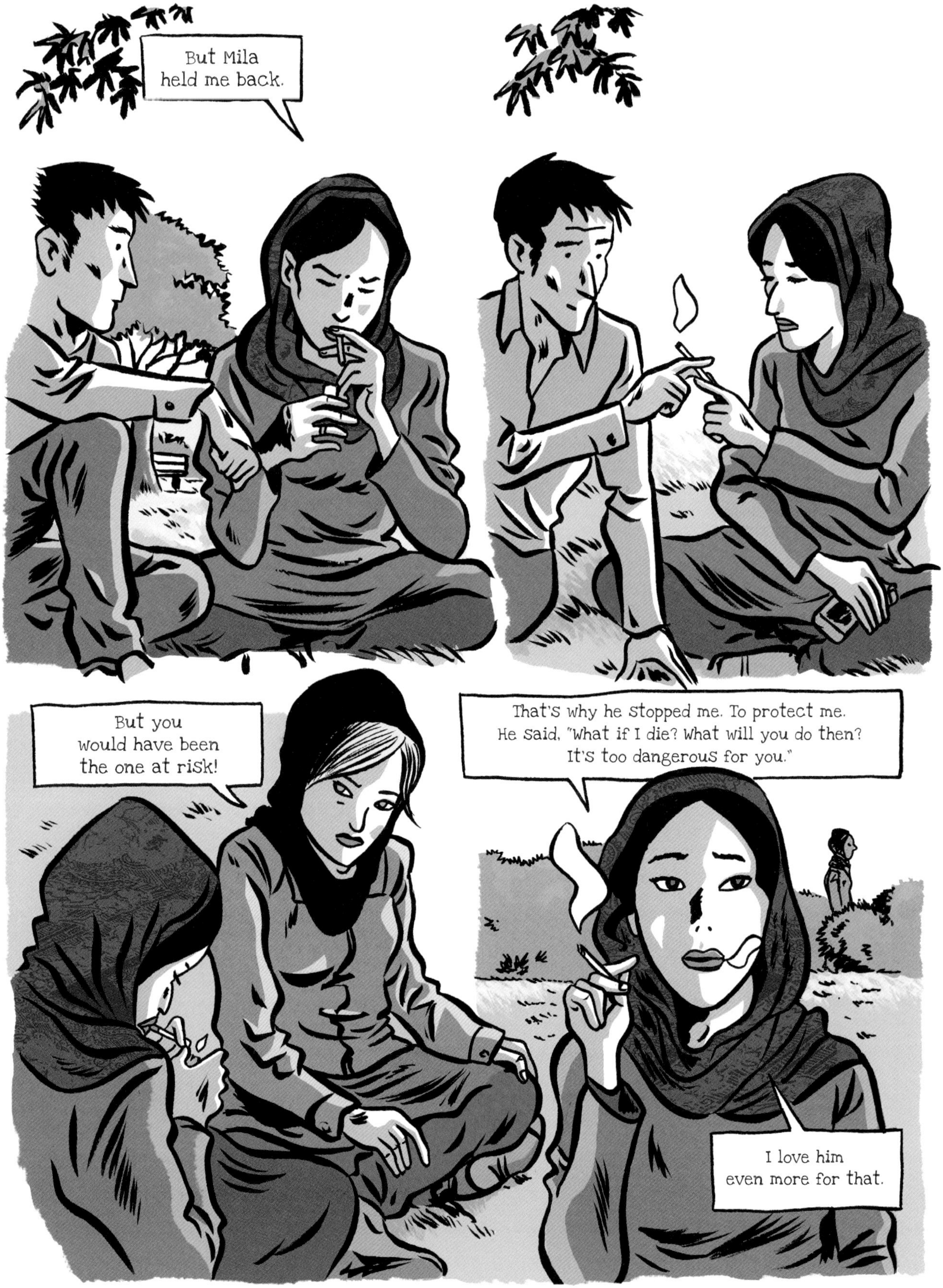
But Mila held me back.
But you would have been the one at risk!
That's why he stopped me. To protect me. He said, "What if I die? What will you do then? It's too dangerous for you."
I love him even more for that.

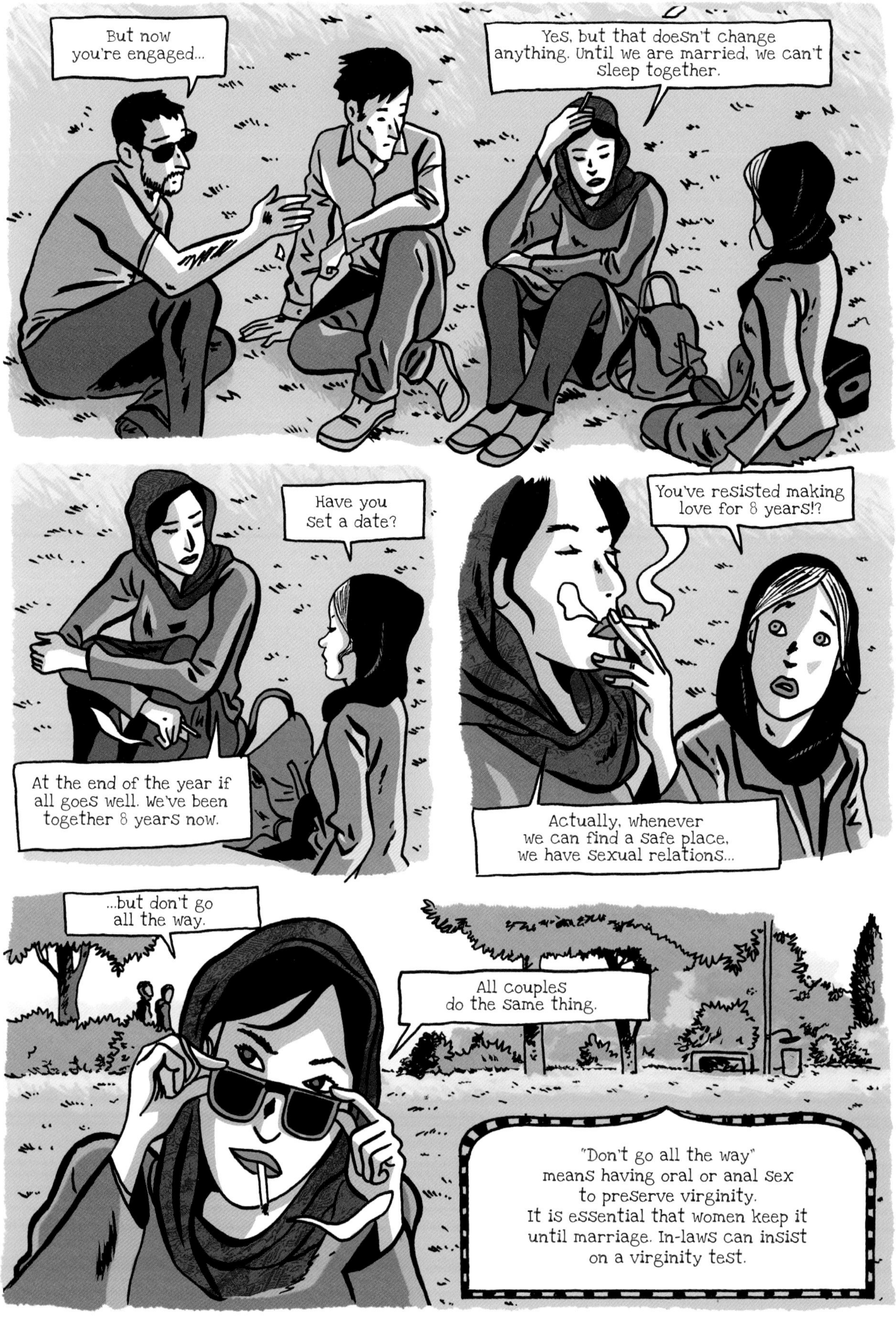
But now you're engaged...
Yes, but that doesn't change anything. Until we are married, we can't sleep together.
Have you set a date?
At the end of the year if all goes well. We've been together 8 years now.
You've resisted making love for 8 years!?
Actually, whenever we can find a safe place, we have sexual relations...
...but don't go all the way.
All couples do the same thing.
"Don't go all the way" means having oral or anal sex to preserve virginity. It is essential that women keep it until marriage. In-laws can insist on a virginity test.

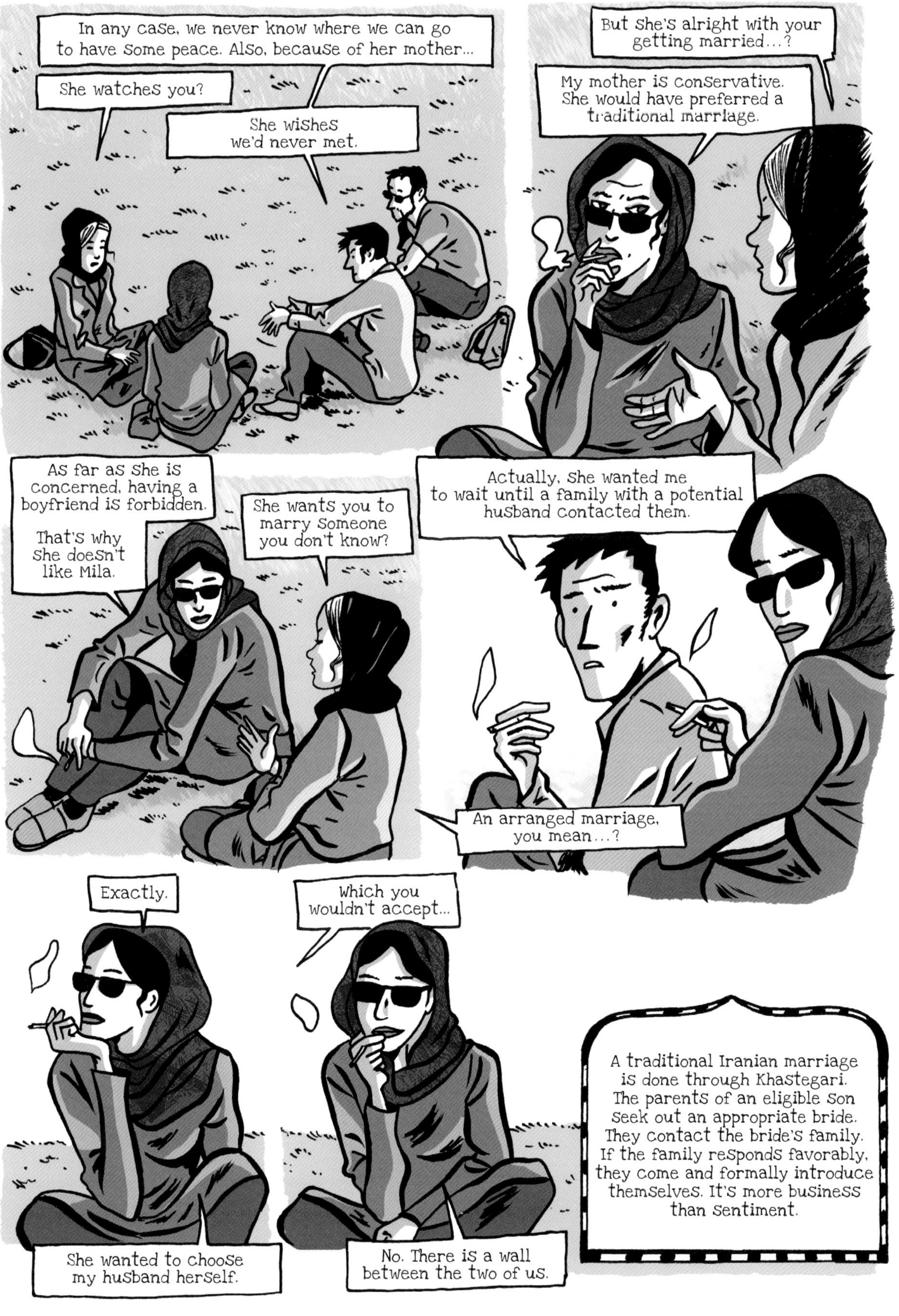
In any case, we never know where we can go to have some peace. Also, because of her mother...
She watches you?
She wishes we'd never met.
But she's alright with your getting married...?
My mother is conservative. She would have preferred a traditional marriage.
As far as she is concerned, having a boyfriend is forbidden.
That's why she doesn't like Mila.
She wants you to marry someone you don't know?
Actually, she wanted me to wait until a family with a potential husband contacted them.
An arranged marriage, you mean...?
Exactly.
She wanted to choose my husband herself.
Which you wouldn't accept...
No. There is a wall between the two of us.
A traditional Iranian marriage is done through Khastegari. The parents of an eligible son seek out an appropriate bride. They contact the bride's family. If the family responds favorably, they come and formally introduce themselves. It's more business than sentiment.

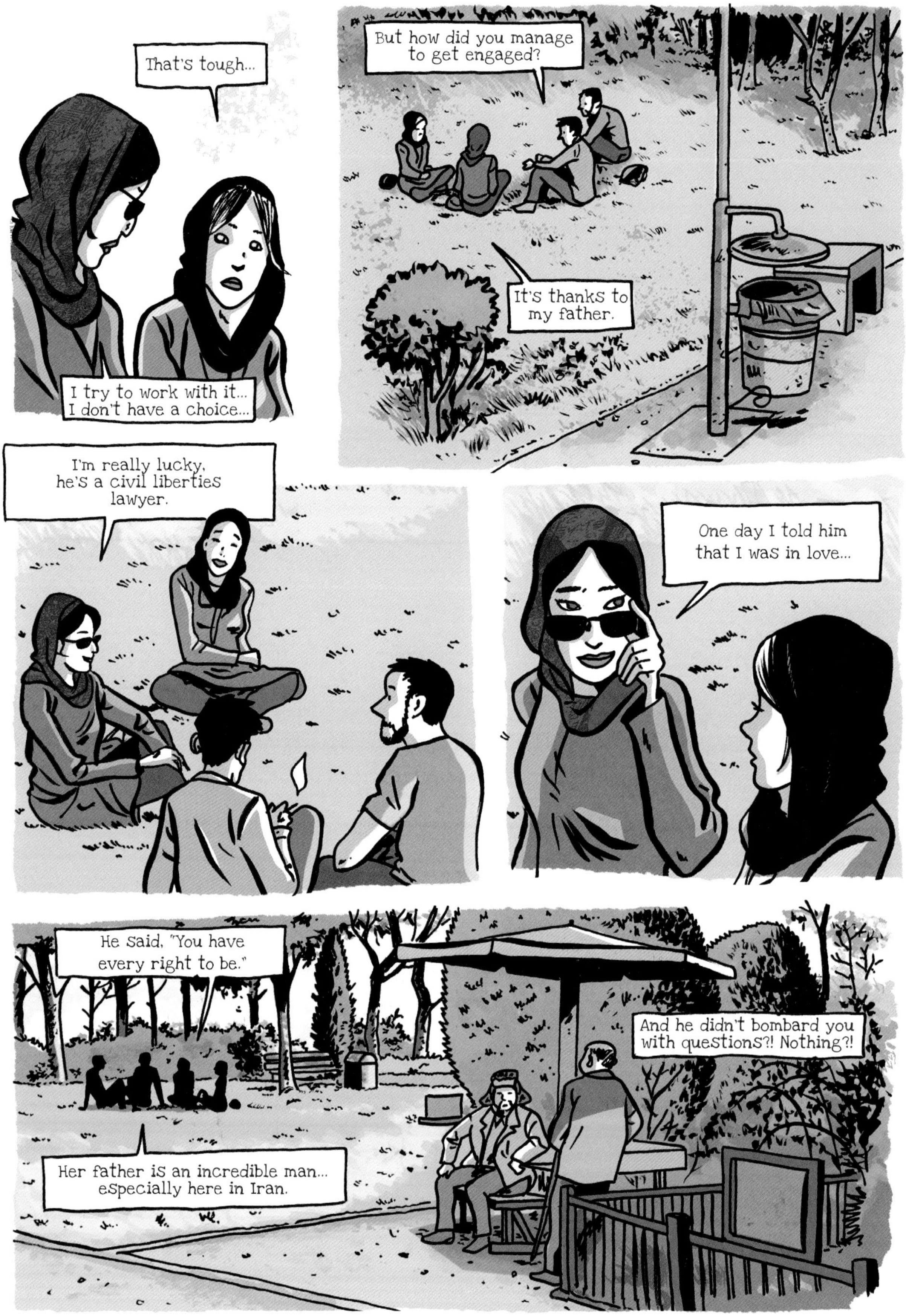
That's tough...
I try to work with it...
I don't have a choice...
But how did you manage to get engaged?
It's thanks to my father.
I'm really lucky, he's a civil liberties lawyer.
One day I told him that I was in love...
He said, "You have every right to be."
Her father is an incredible man... especially here in Iran.
And he didn't bombard you with questions?! Nothing?!

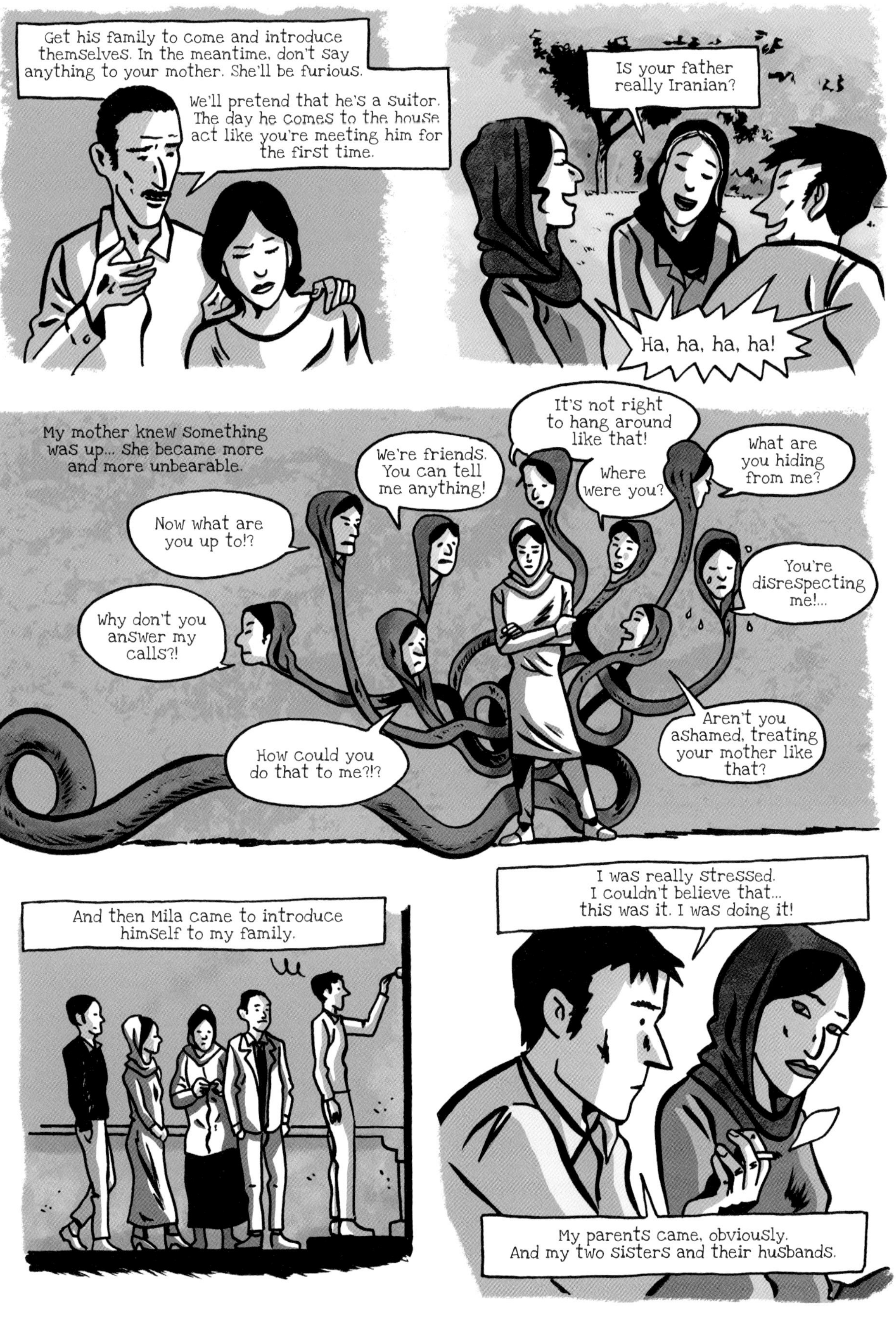
Get his family to come and introduce themselves. In the meantime, don't say anything to your mother. She'll be furious.
We'll pretend that he's a suitor. The day he comes to the house act like you're meeting him for the first time.
Is your father really Iranian?
Ha, ha, ha, ha!
My mother knew something was up... she became more and more unbearable.
Now what are you up to!?
Why don't you answer my calls?!
We're friends. You can tell me anything!
It's not right to hang around like that!
Where were you?
What are you hiding from me?
You're disrespecting me!...
How could you do that to me?!?
Aren't you ashamed, treating your mother like that?
And then Mila came to introduce himself to my family.
I was really stressed. I couldn't believe that... this was it. I was doing it!
My parents came, obviously. And my two sisters and their husbands.

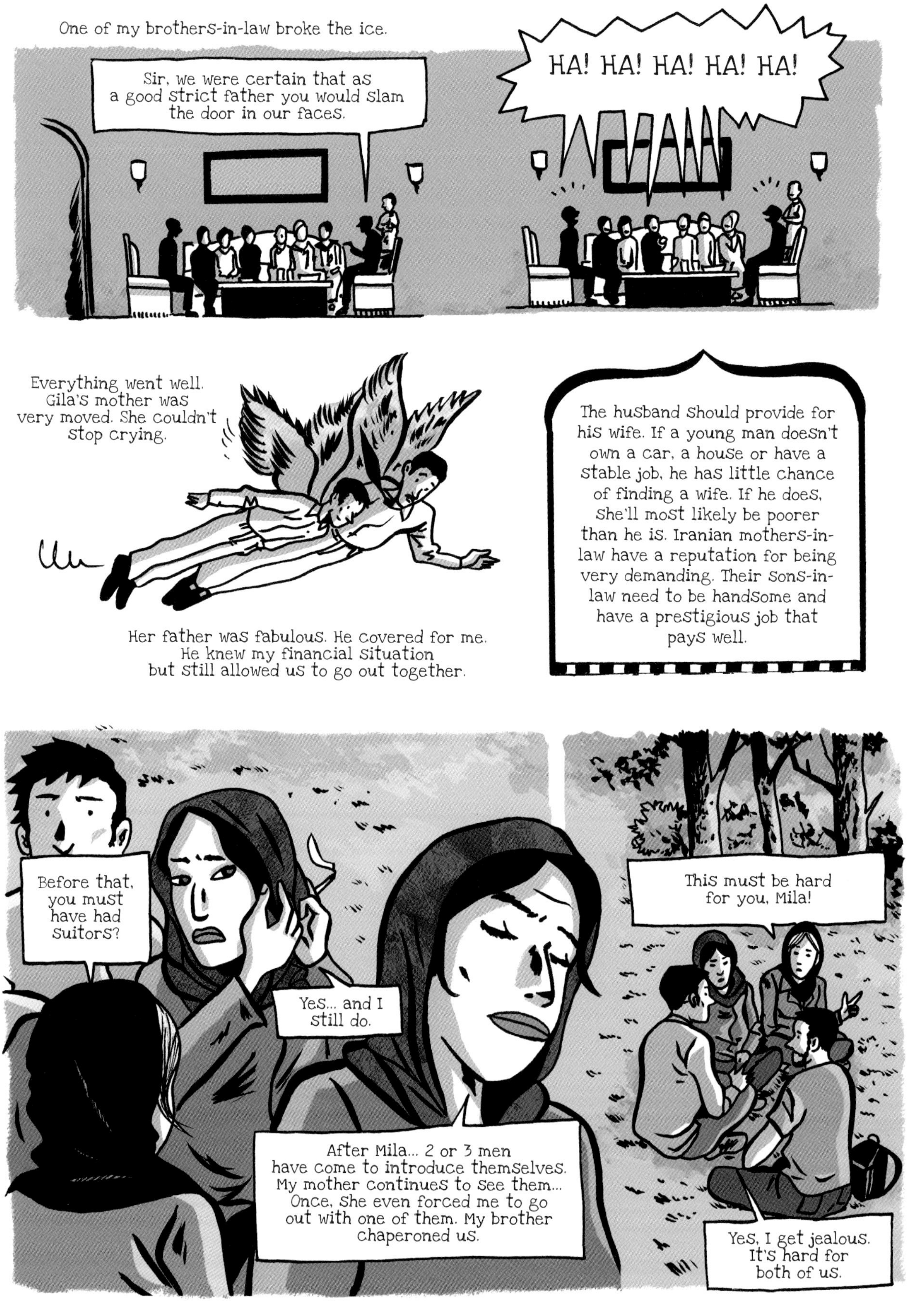
One of my brothers-in-law broke the ice.
Sir, we were certain that as a good strict father you would slam the door in our faces.
HA! HA! HA! HA! HA!
Everything went well. Gila's mother was very moved. She couldn't stop crying.
Her father was fabulous. He covered for me. He knew my financial situation but still allowed us to go out together.
The husband should provide for his wife. If a young man doesn't own a car, a house or have a stable job, he has little chance of finding a wife. If he does, she'll most likely be poorer than he is. Iranian mothers-in-law have a reputation for being very demanding. Their sons-in-law need to be handsome and have a prestigious job that pays well.
Before that, you must have had suitors?
Yes... and I still do.
After Mila... 2 or 3 men have come to introduce themselves. My mother continues to see them... Once, she even forced me to go out with one of them. My brother chaperoned us.
This must be hard for you, Mila!
Yes, I get jealous. It's hard for both of us.

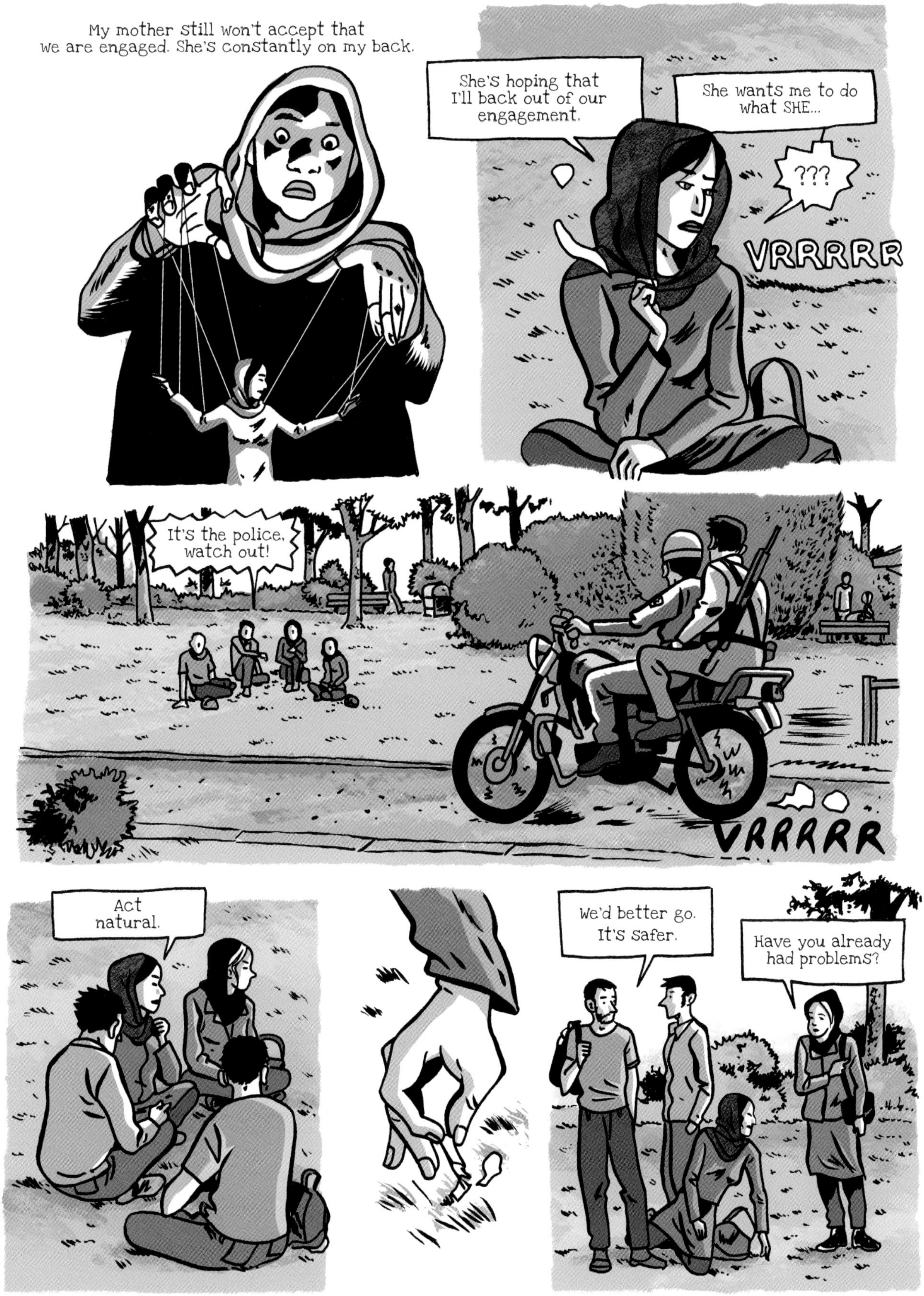

My mother still won't accept that we are engaged. She's constantly on my back.
She's hoping that I'll back out of our engagement.
She wants me to do what SHE...
???
VRRRRR
It's the police, watch out!
VRRRRR
Act natural.
We'd better go. It's safer.
Have you already had problems?

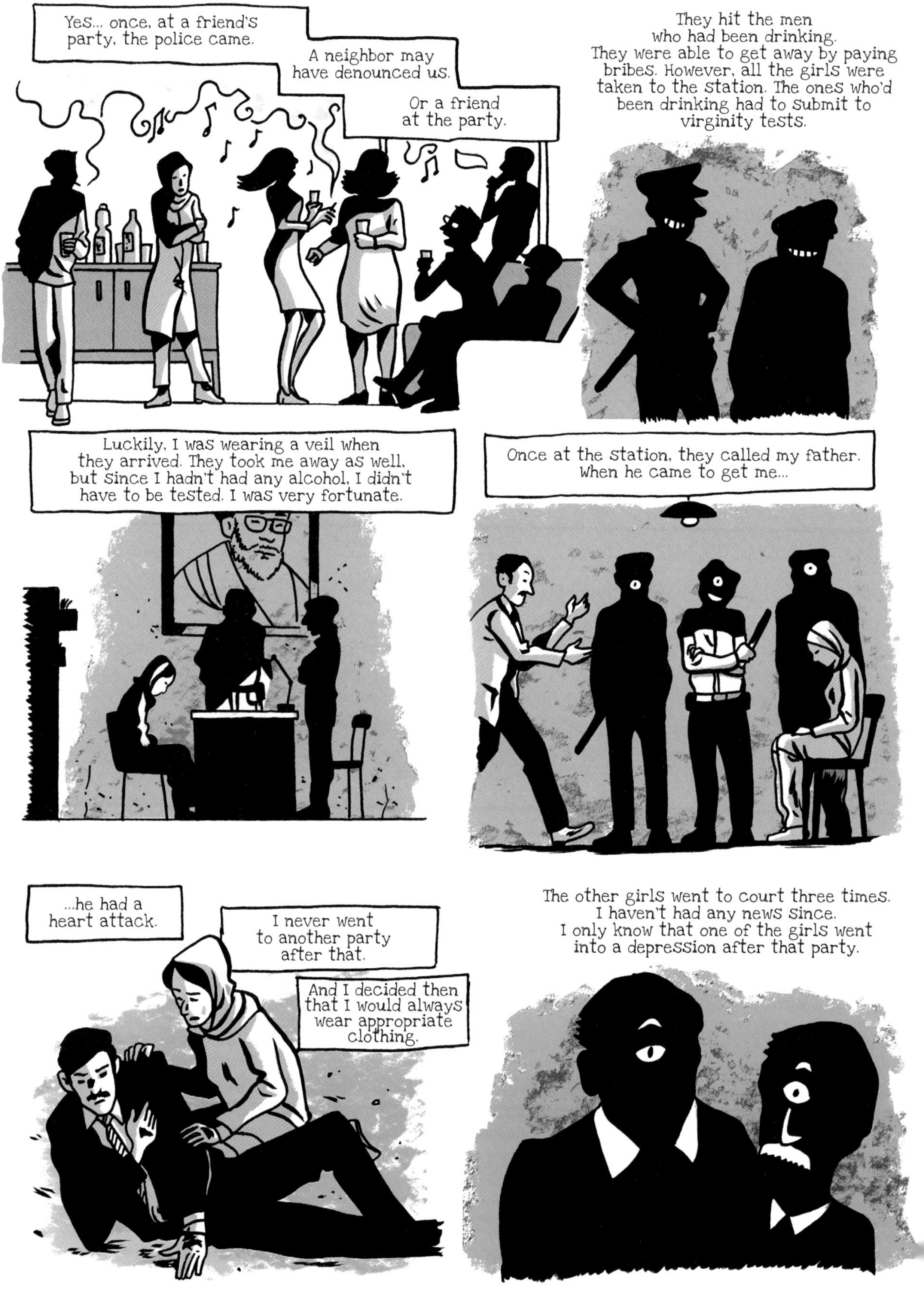

Yes... once, at a friend's party, the police came.
A neighbor may have denounced us.
Or a friend at the party.
They hit the men who had been drinking. They were able to get away by paying bribes. However, all the girls were taken to the station. The ones who'd been drinking had to submit to virginity tests.
Luckily, I was wearing a veil when they arrived. They took me away as well, but since I hadn't had any alcohol, I didn't have to be tested. I was very fortunate.
Once at the station, they called my father. When he came to get me...
...he had a heart attack.
I never went to another party after that.
And I decided then that I would always wear appropriate clothing.
The other girls went to court three times. I haven't had any news since. I only know that one of the girls went into a depression after that party.

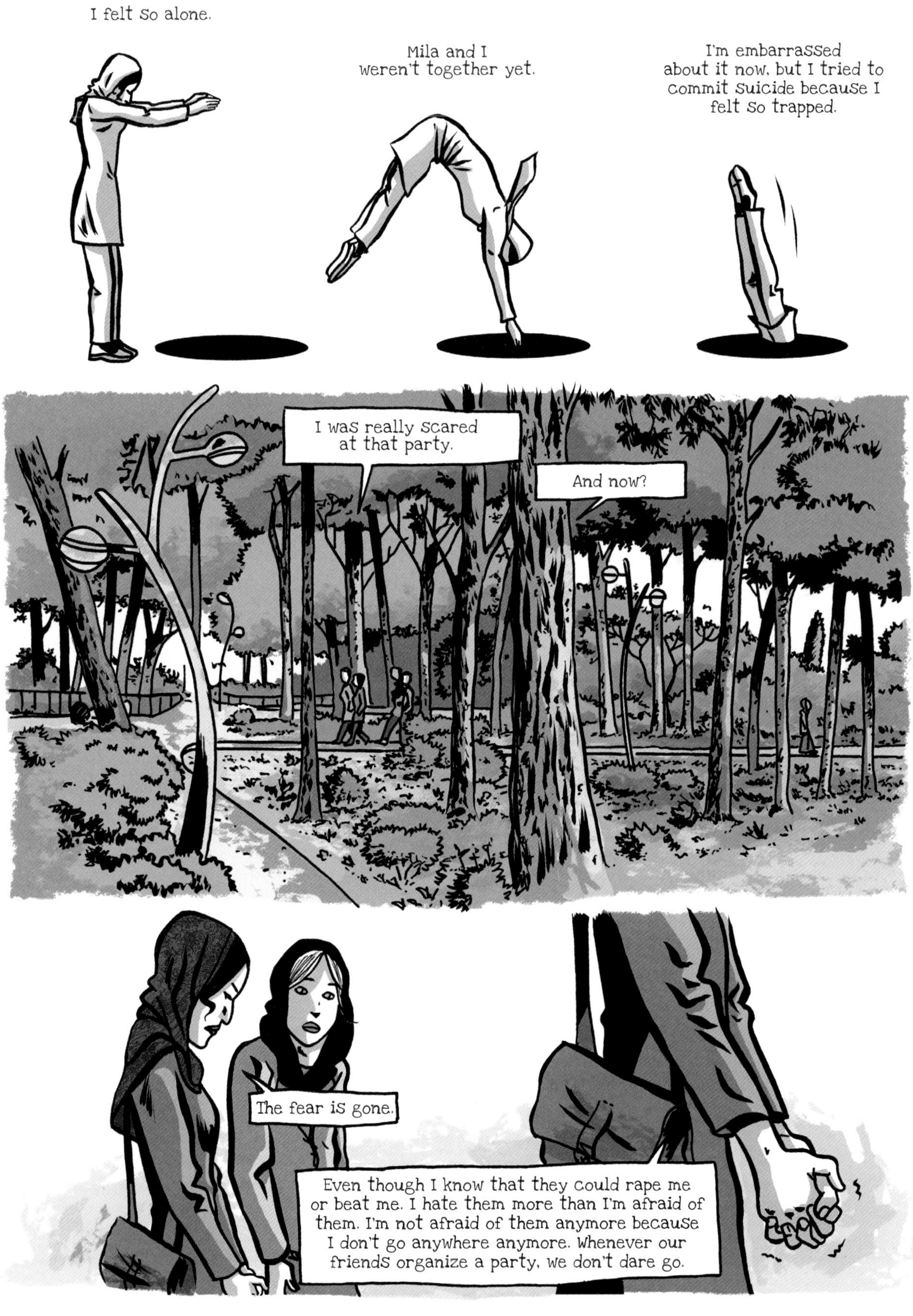
I felt so alone.
Mila and I weren't together yet.
I'm embarrassed about it now, but I tried to commit suicide because I felt so trapped.
I was really scared at that party.
And now?
The fear is gone.
Even though I know that they could rape me or beat me. I hate them more than I'm afraid of them. I'm not afraid of them anymore because I don't go anywhere anymore. Whenever our friends organize a party, we don't dare go.

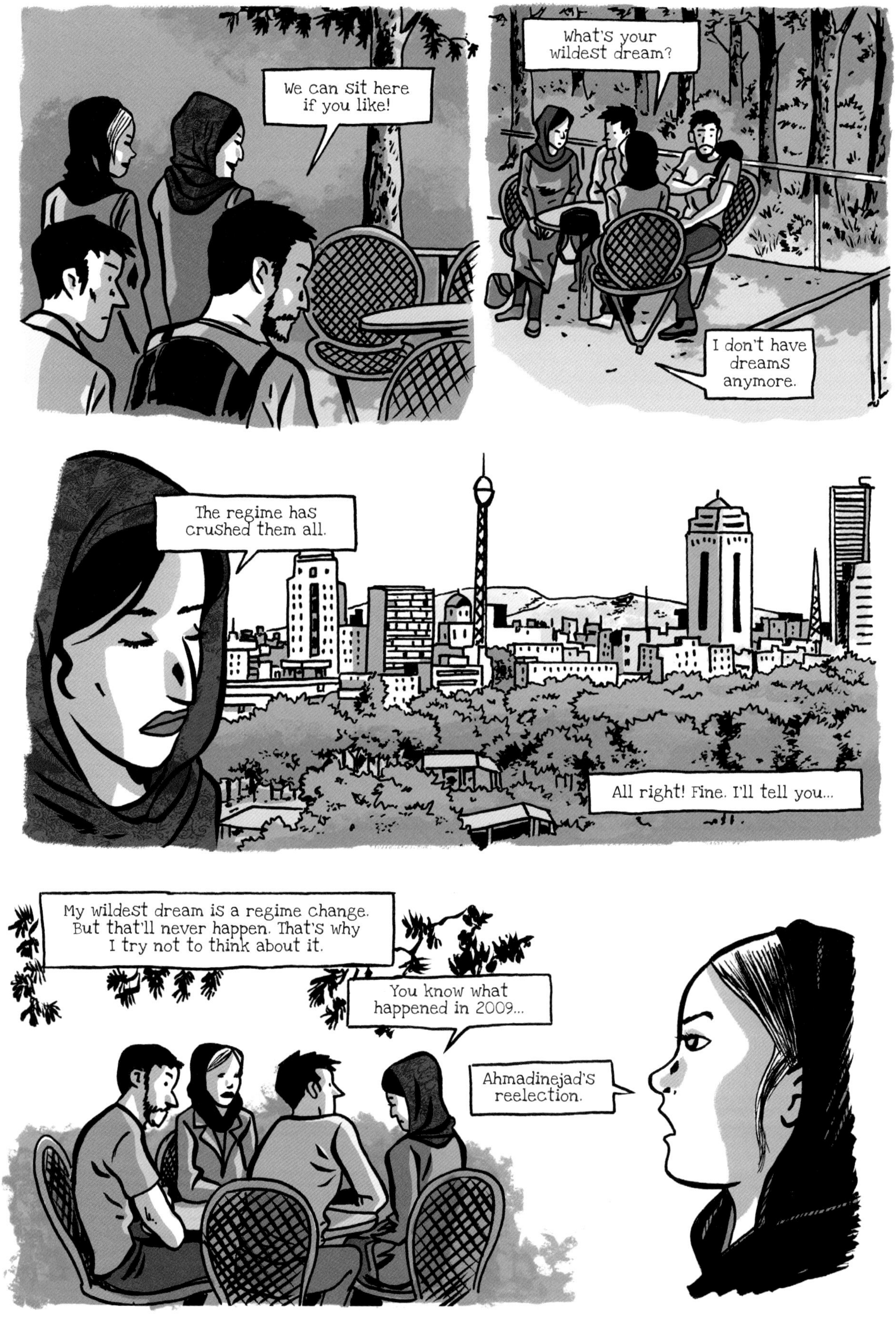
We can sit here if you like!
What's your wildest dream?
I don't have dreams anymore.
The regime has crushed them all.
All right! Fine. I'll tell you...
My wildest dream is a regime change. But that'll never happen. That's why I try not to think about it.
You know what happened in 2009...
Ahmadinejad's reelection.

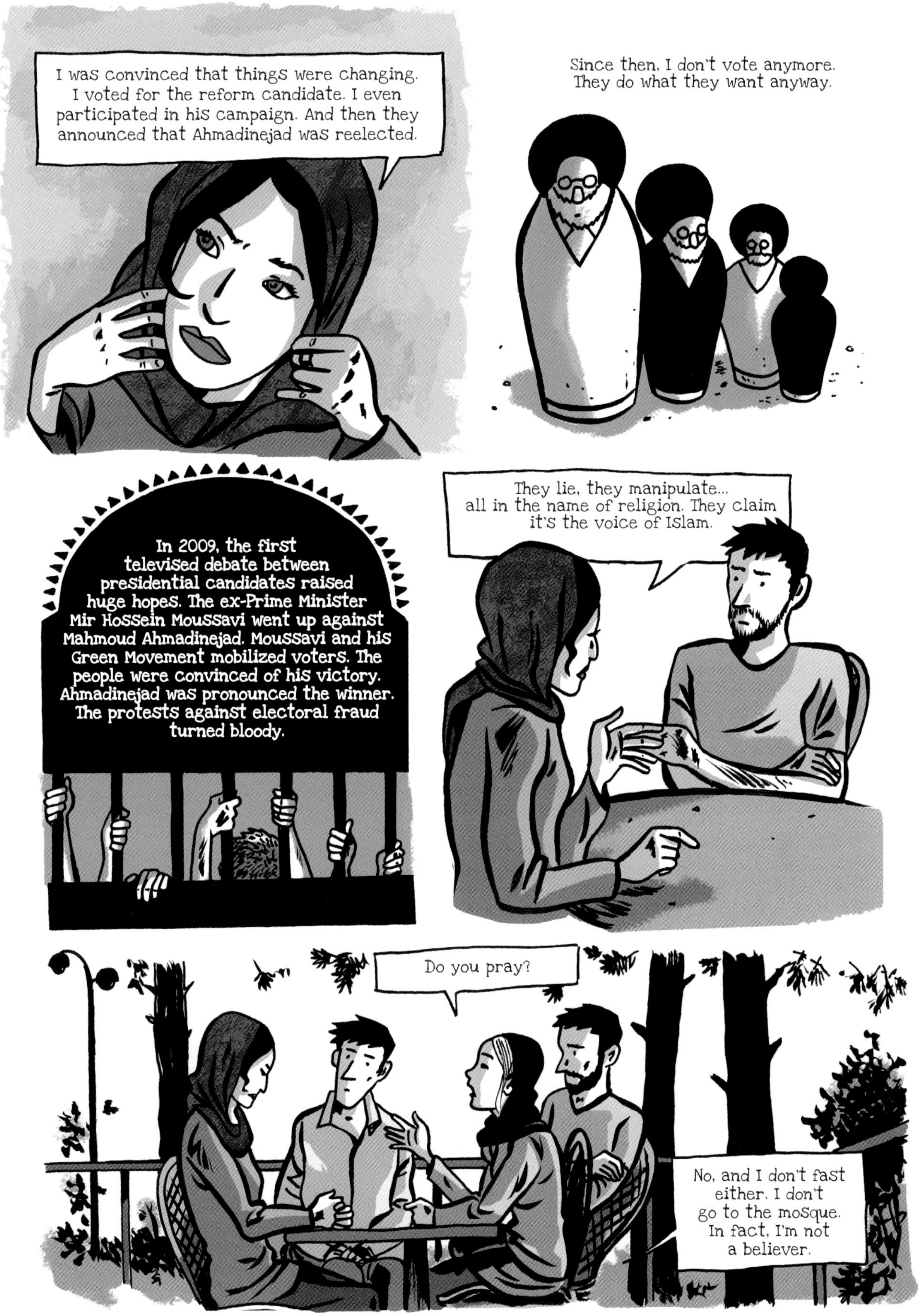
I was convinced that things were changing. I voted for the reform candidate. I even participated in his campaign. And then they announced that Ahmadinejad was reelected.
Since then, I don't vote anymore. They do what they want anyway.
In 2009, the first televised debate between presidential candidates raised huge hopes. The ex-Prime Minister Mir Hossein Moussavi went up against Mahmoud Ahmadinejad. Moussavi and his Green Movement mobilized voters. The people were convinced of his victory. Ahmadinejad was pronounced the winner. The protests against electoral fraud turned bloody.
They lie, they manipulate... all in the name of religion. They claim it's the voice of Islam.
Do you pray?
No, and I don't fast either. I don't go to the mosque. In fact, I'm not a believer.

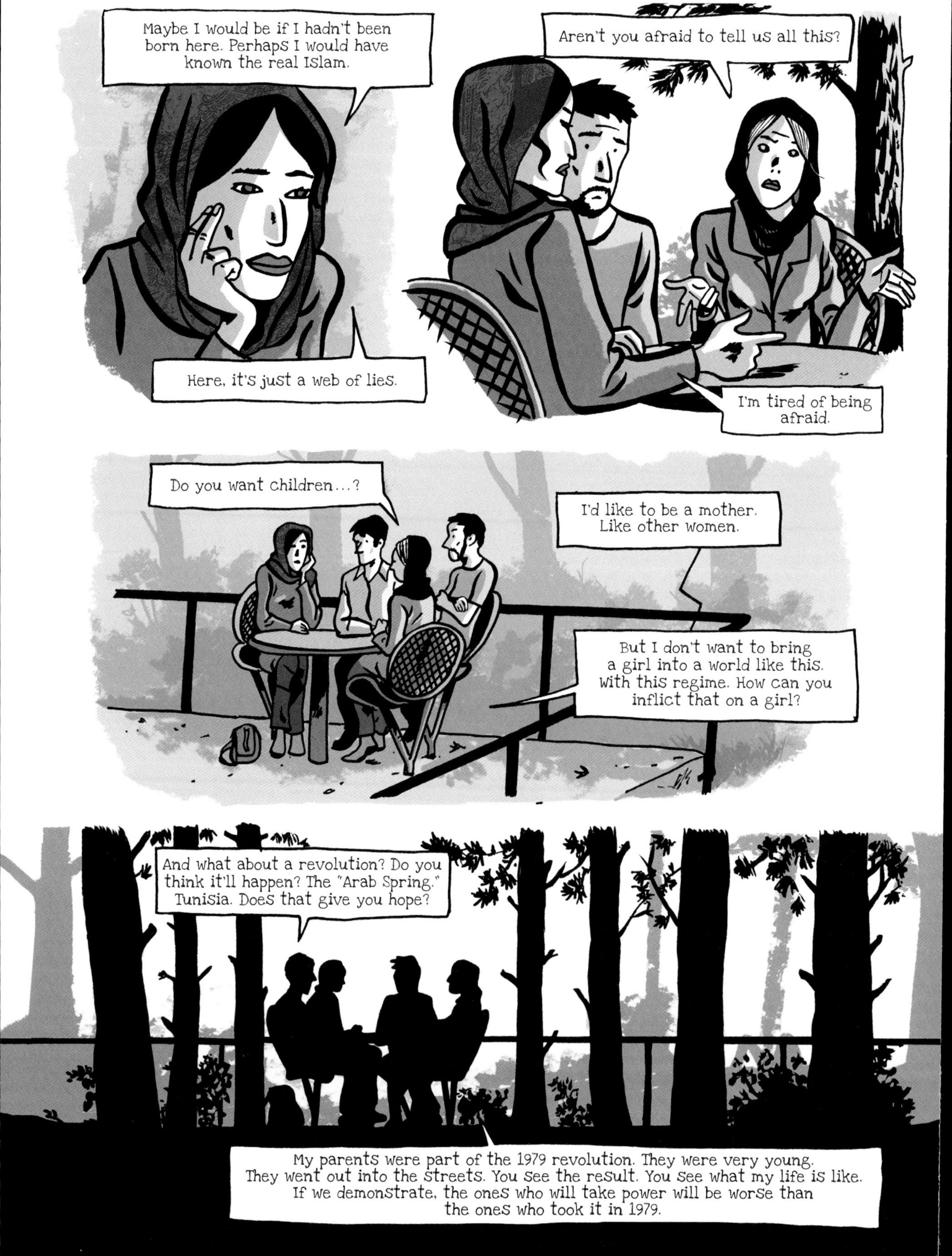

Maybe I would be if I hadn't been born here. Perhaps I would have known the real Islam.
Here, it's just a web of lies.
Aren't you afraid to tell us all this?
I'm tired of being afraid.
Do you want children...?
I'd like to be a mother. Like other women.
But I don't want to bring a girl into a world like this. With this regime. How can you inflict that on a girl?
And what about a revolution? Do you think it'll happen? The "Arab Spring." Tunisia. Does that give you hope?
My parents were part of the 1979 revolution. They were very young. They went out into the streets. You see the result. You see what my life is like. If we demonstrate, the ones who will take power will be worse than the ones who took it in 1979.

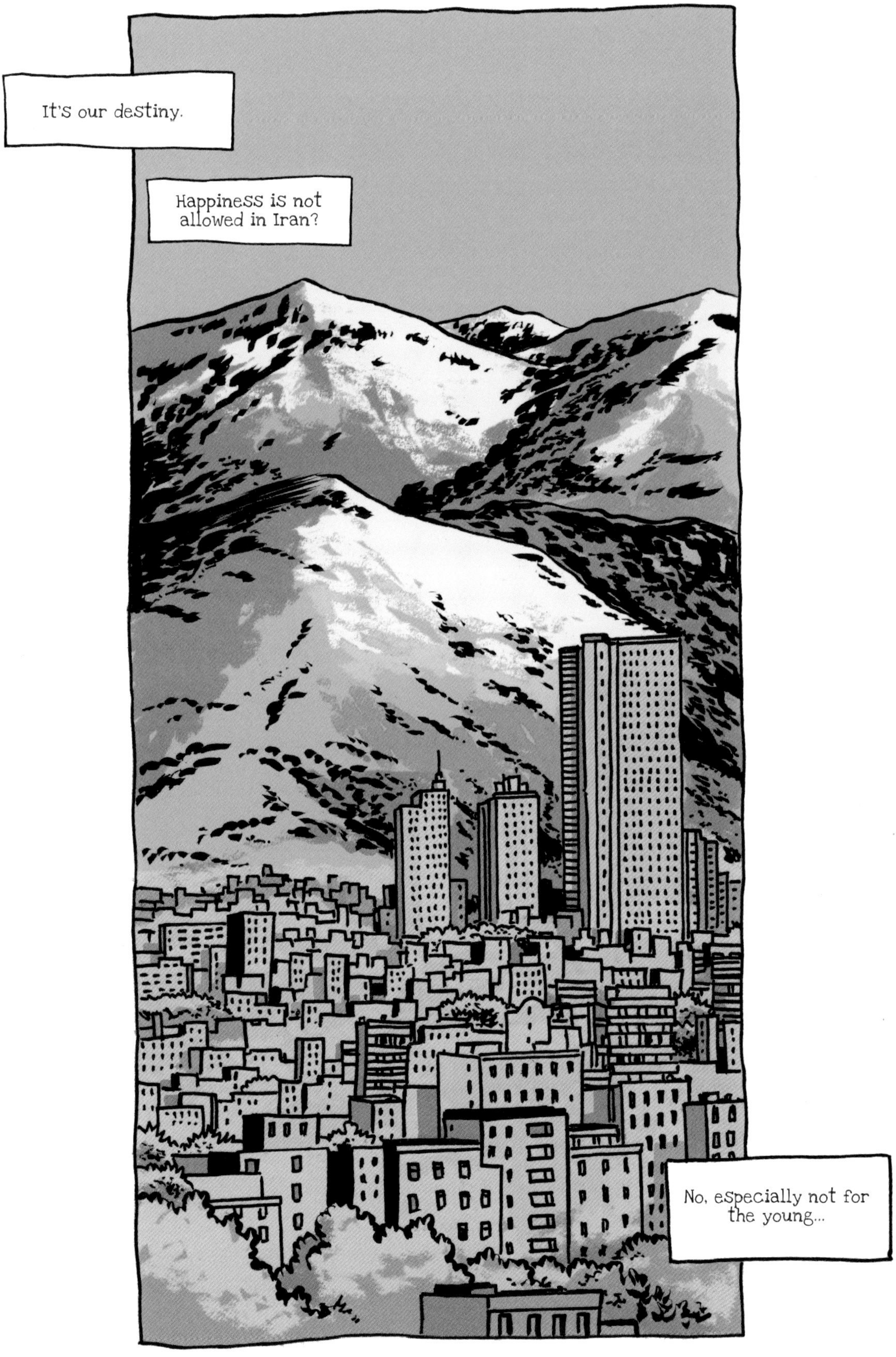
It's our destiny.
Happiness is not allowed in Iran?
No, especially not for the young...

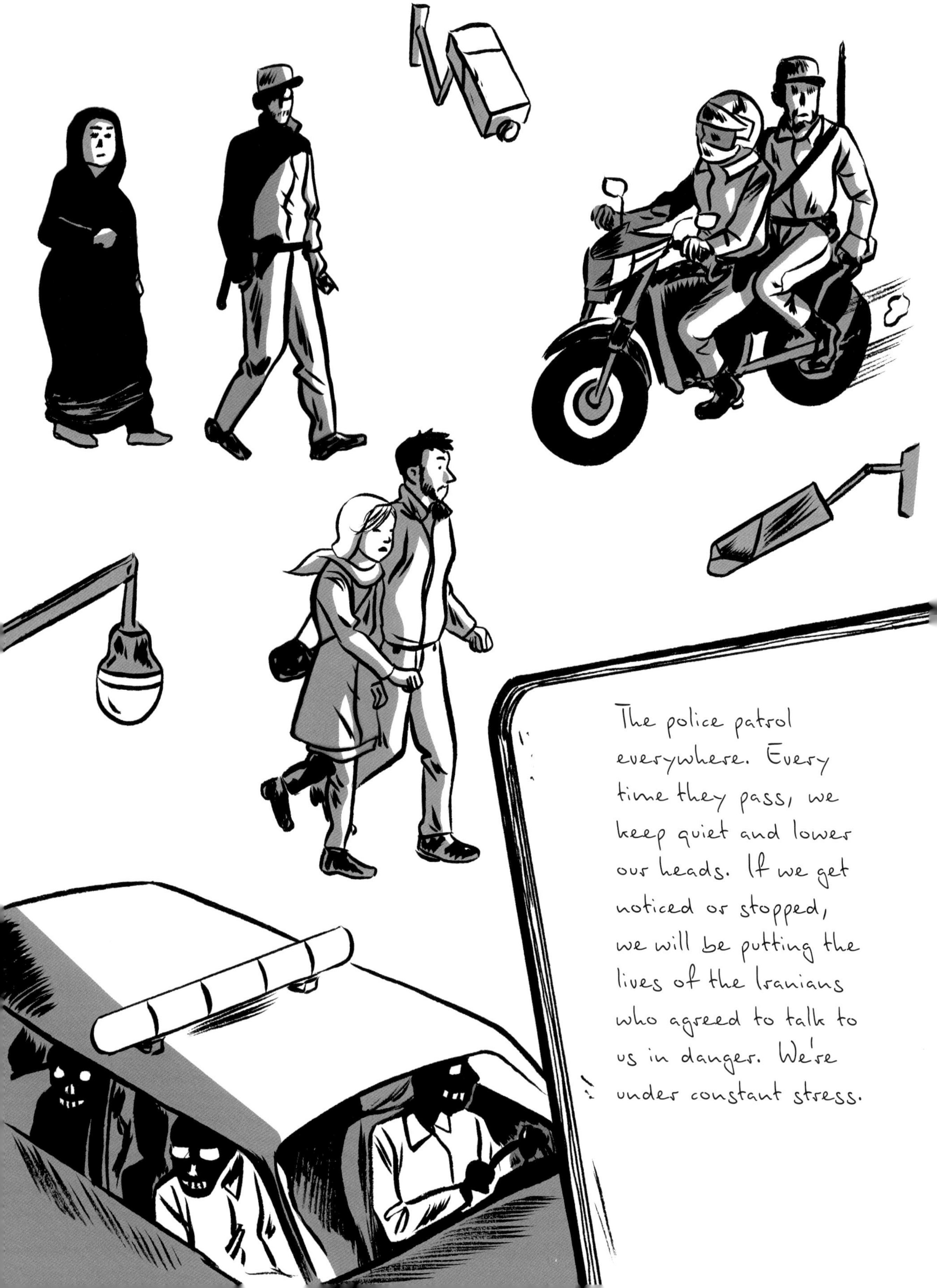
The police patrol everywhere. Every time they pass, we keep quiet and lower our heads. If we get noticed or stopped, we will be putting the lives of the Iranians who agreed to talk to us in danger. We're under constant stress.

تهیه غذای
فارسی
فارسی شعبه ندارد

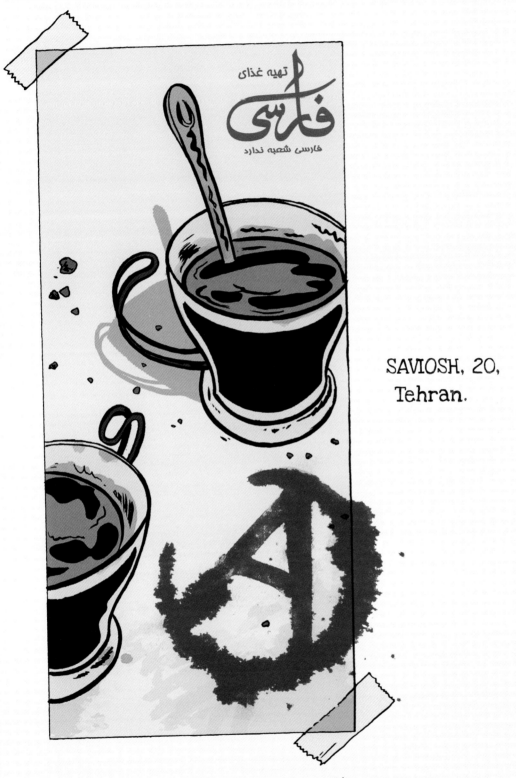

SAVIOSH, 20,
Tehran.

Saviosh lives between two worlds. He is a waiter in an upscale café in the north of Tehran but lives in a working-class district in the south of the city. If he hadn't been born in Iran, he would have been a musician.

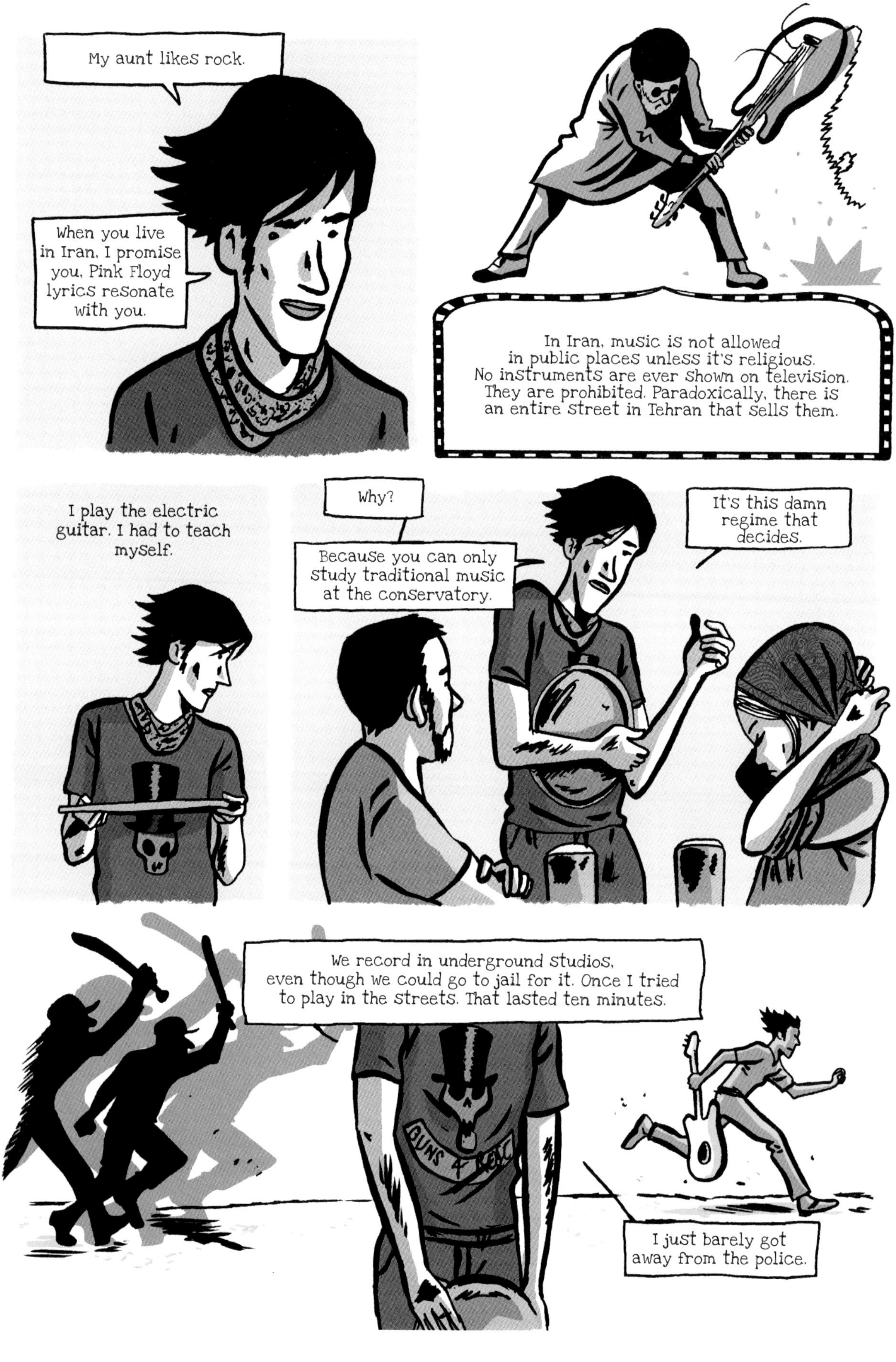
My aunt likes rock.
When you live in Iran, I promise you, Pink Floyd lyrics resonate with you.
In Iran, music is not allowed in public places unless it's religious. No instruments are ever shown on television. They are prohibited. Paradoxically, there is an entire street in Tehran that sells them.
I play the electric guitar. I had to teach myself.
Why?
Because you can only study traditional music at the conservatory.
It's this damn regime that decides.
We record in underground studios, even though we could go to jail for it. Once I tried to play in the streets. That lasted ten minutes.
I just barely got away from the police.

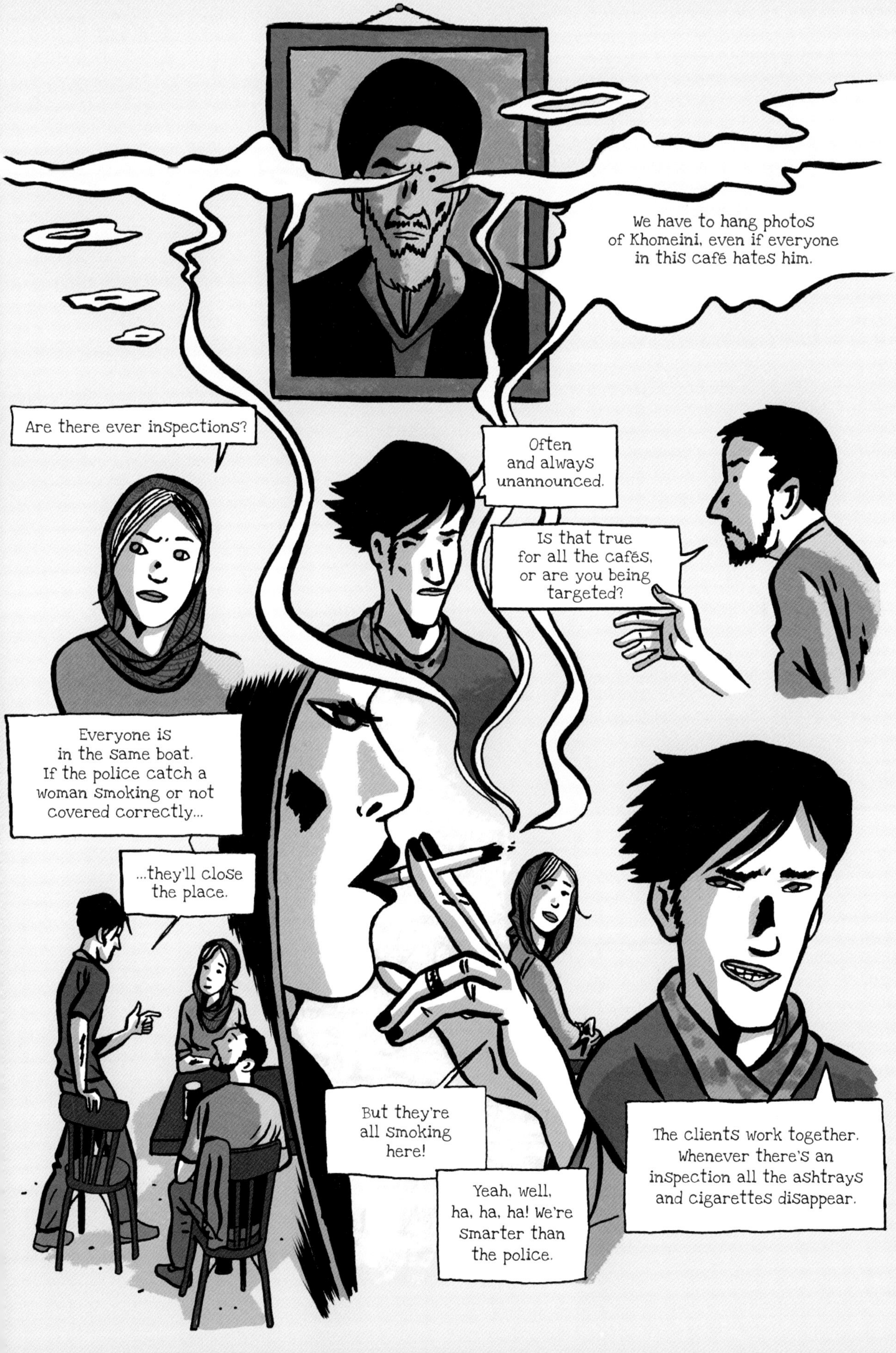
We have to hang photos of Khomeini, even if everyone in this café hates him.
Are there ever inspections?
Often and always unannounced.
Is that true for all the cafés, or are you being targeted?
Everyone is in the same boat. If the police catch a woman smoking or not covered correctly...
...they'll close the place.
But they're all smoking here!
The clients work together. Whenever there's an inspection all the ashtrays and cigarettes disappear.
Yeah, well, ha, ha, ha! We're smarter than the police.

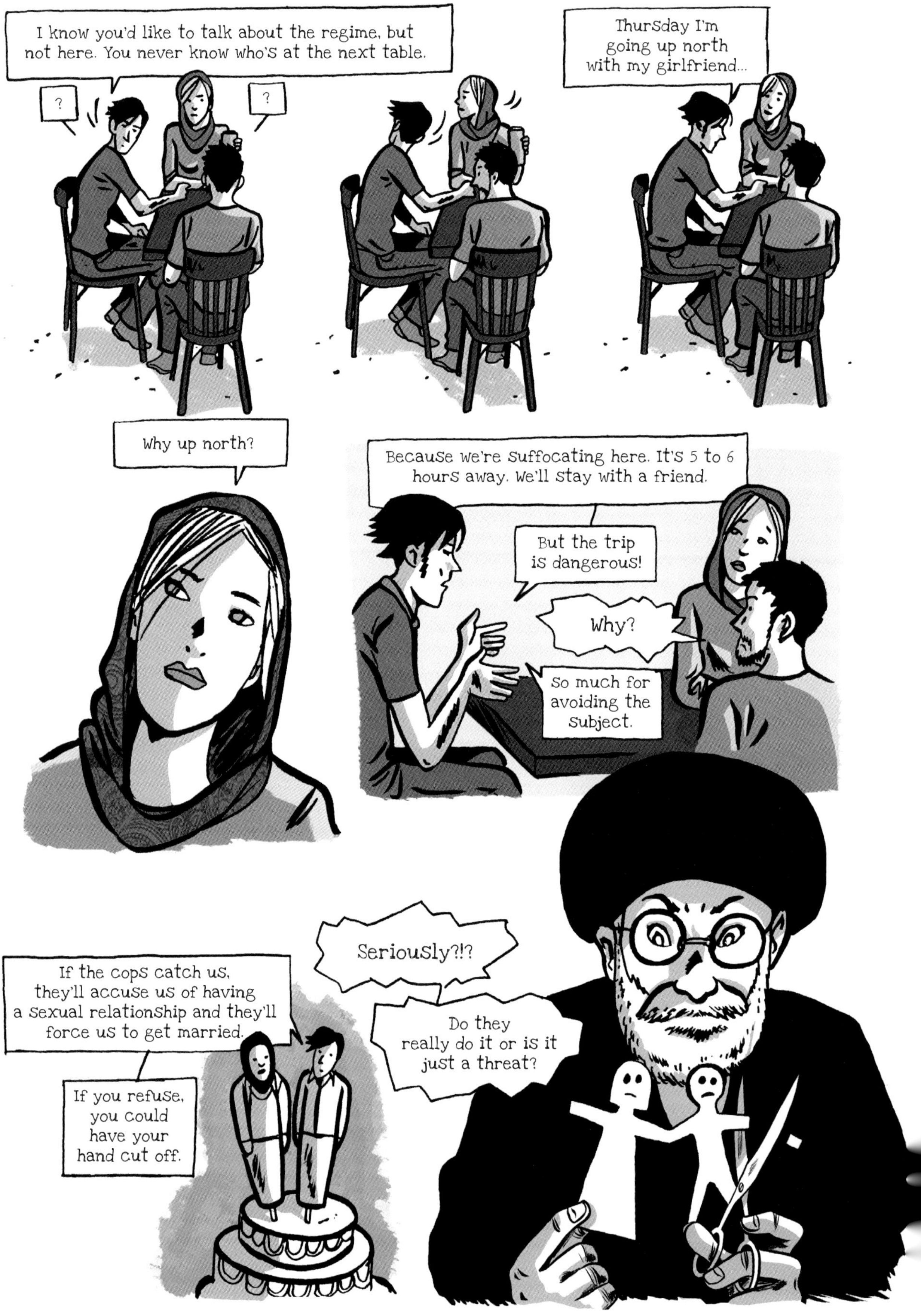
I know you'd like to talk about the regime, but not here. You never know who's at the next table.
?
?
Thursday I'm going up north with my girlfriend...
Why up north?
Because we're suffocating here. It's 5 to 6 hours away. We'll stay with a friend.
But the trip is dangerous!
Why?
So much for avoiding the subject.
If the cops catch us, they'll accuse us of having a sexual relationship and they'll force us to get married.
If you refuse, you could have your hand cut off.
Seriously?!?
Do they really do it or is it just a threat?

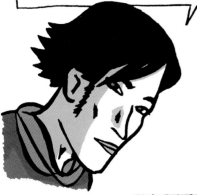

We have friends who were stopped. To be released, they had to get married on the spot.

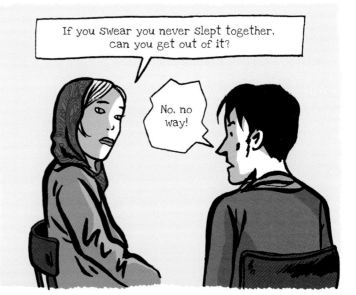

If you swear you never slept together, can you get out of it?

No, no way!

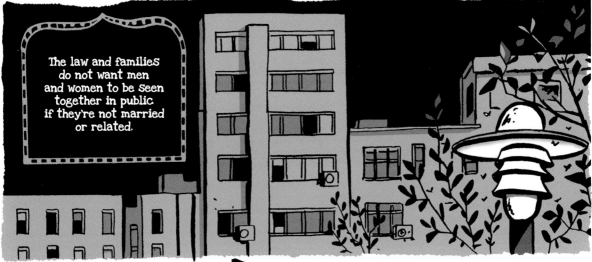

The law and families do not want men and women to be seen together in public if they're not married or related.

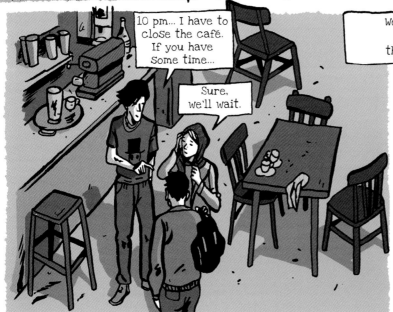

10 pm... I have to close the café. If you have some time...

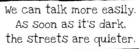

Sure, we'll wait.

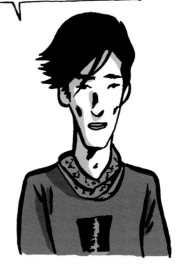

We can talk more easily. As soon as it's dark, the streets are quieter.

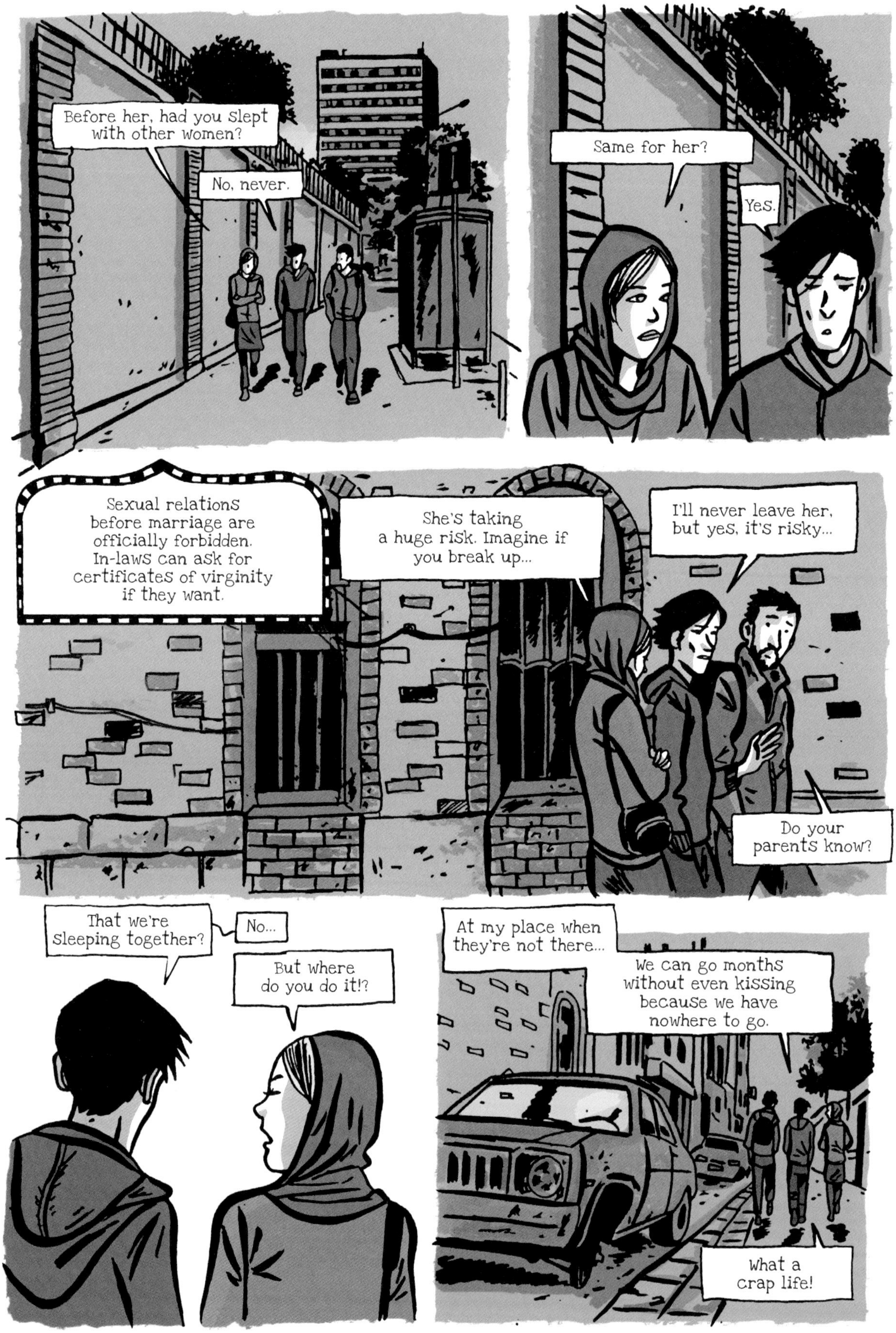
Before her, had you slept with other women?
No, never.
Same for her?
Yes.
Sexual relations before marriage are officially forbidden. In-laws can ask for certificates of virginity if they want.
She's taking a huge risk. Imagine if you break up...
I'll never leave her, but yes, it's risky...
Do your parents know?
That we're sleeping together?
No...
But where do you do it!?
At my place when they're not there...
We can go months without even kissing because we have nowhere to go.
What a crap life!

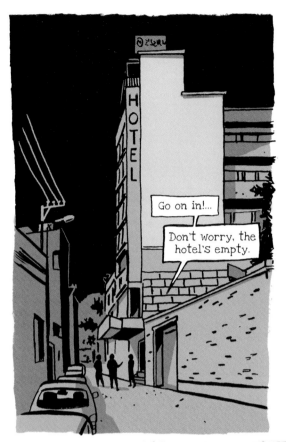

Go on in!...

Don't worry, the hotel's empty.

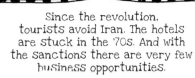

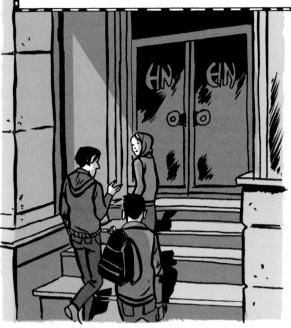

Since the revolution, tourists avoid Iran. The hotels are stuck in the '70s. And with the sanctions there are very few business opportunities.

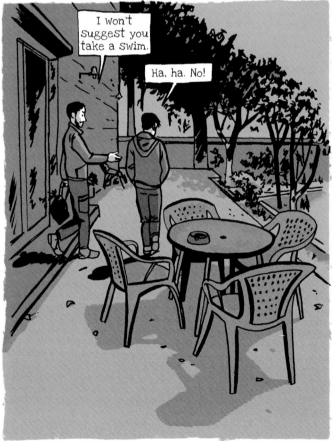

I won't suggest you take a swim.

Ha, ha. No!

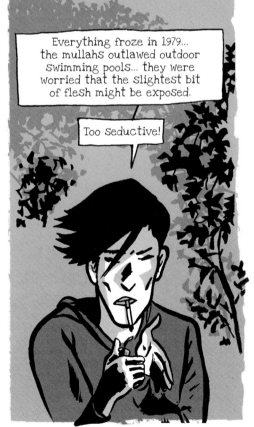

Everything froze in 1979... the mullahs outlawed outdoor swimming pools... they were worried that the slightest bit of flesh might be exposed.

Too seductive!

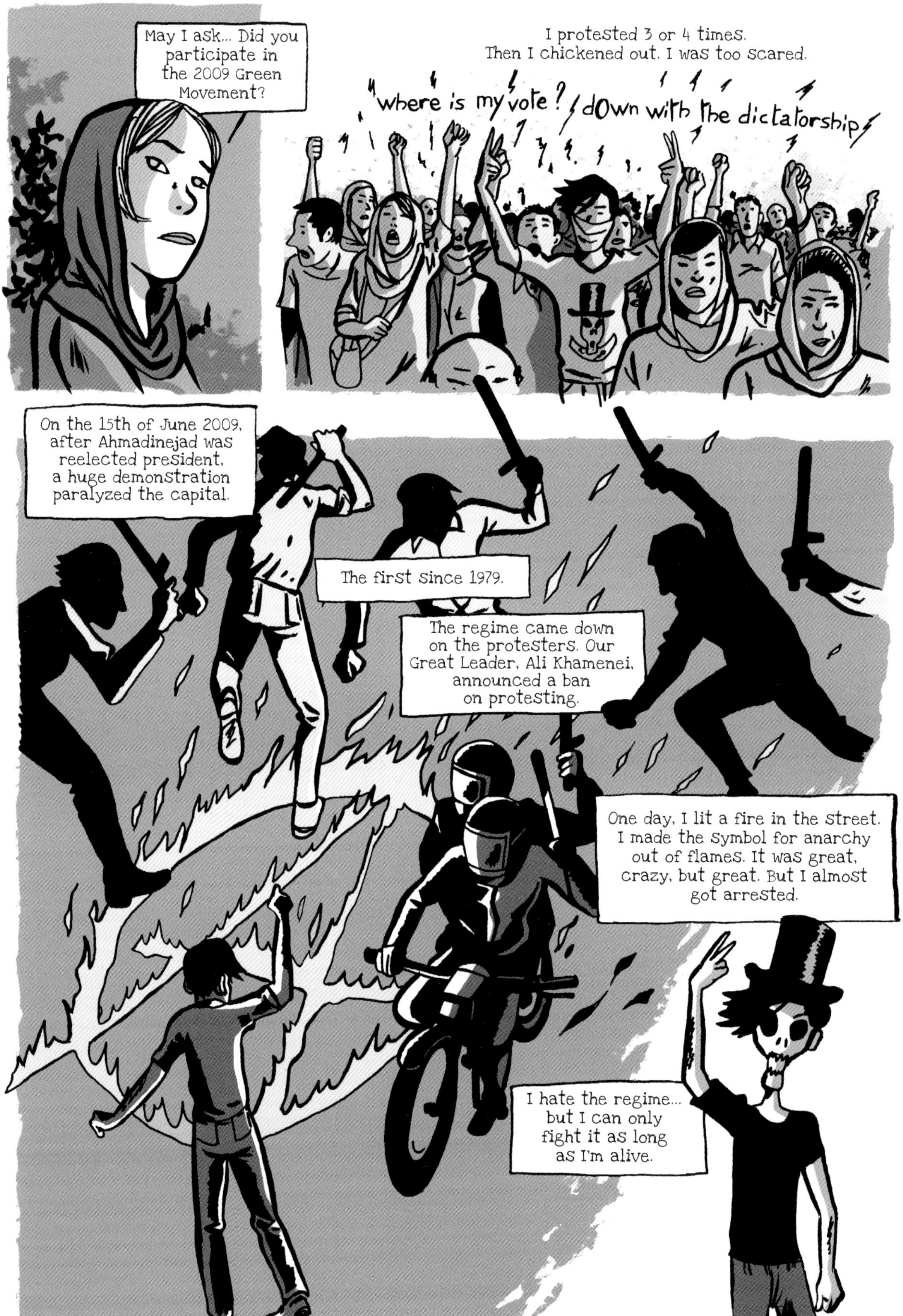
May I ask... Did you participate in the 2009 Green Movement?
I protested 3 or 4 times. Then I chickened out. I was too scared.
where is my vote?
down with the dictatorship
On the 15th of June 2009, after Ahmadinejad was reelected president, a huge demonstration paralyzed the capital.
The first since 1979.
The regime came down on the protesters. Our Great Leader, Ali Khamenei, announced a ban on protesting.
One day, I lit a fire in the street. I made the symbol for anarchy out of flames. It was great, crazy, but great. But I almost got arrested.
I hate the regime... but I can only fight it as long as I'm alive.

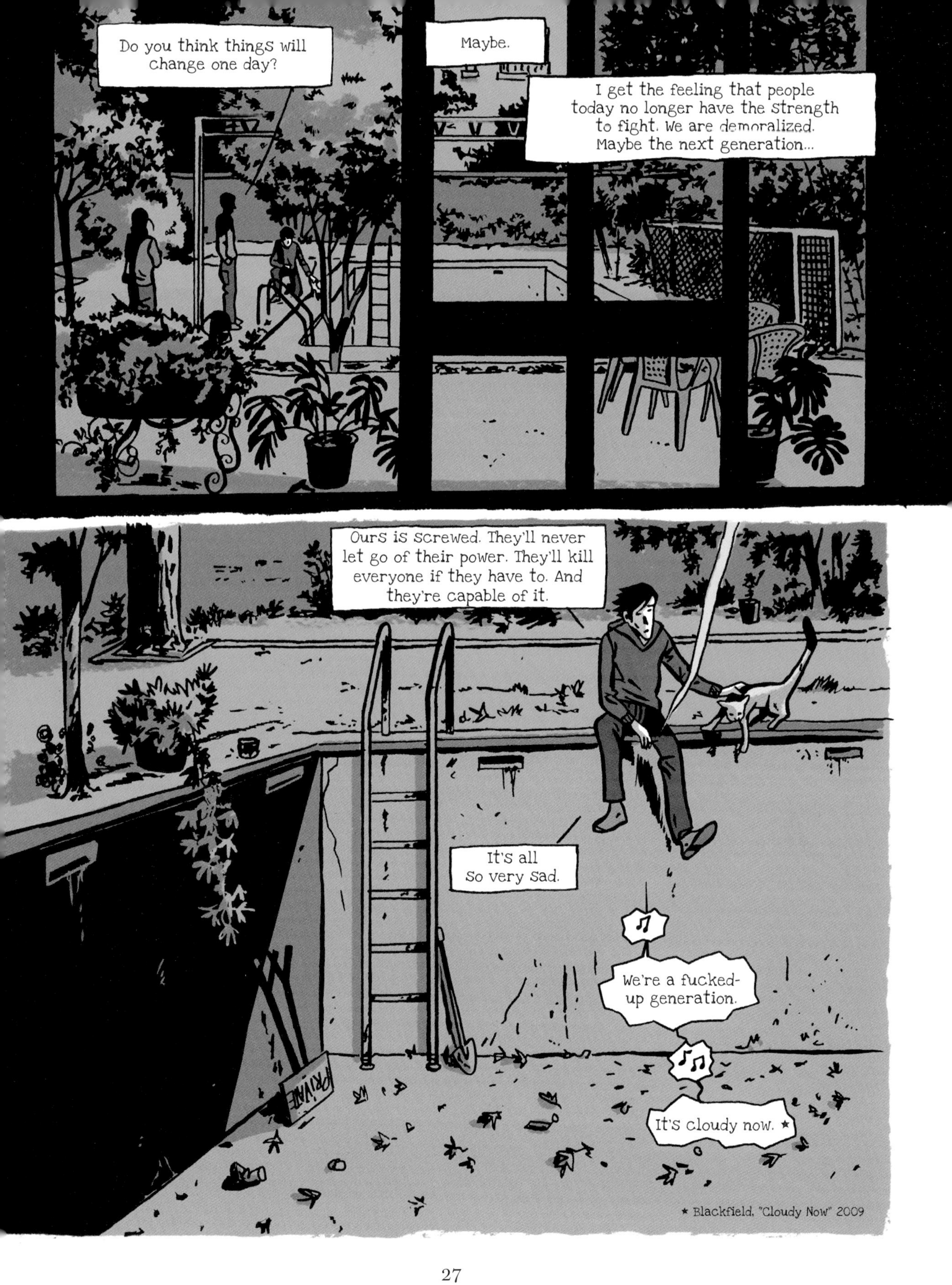
Do you think things will change one day?
Maybe.
I get the feeling that people today no longer have the strength to fight. We are demoralized. Maybe the next generation...
Ours is screwed. They'll never let go of their power. They'll kill everyone if they have to. And they're capable of it.
It's all so very sad.
We're a fucked-up generation.
It's cloudy now. *
PRIVATE
* Blackfield, "Cloudy Now" 2009

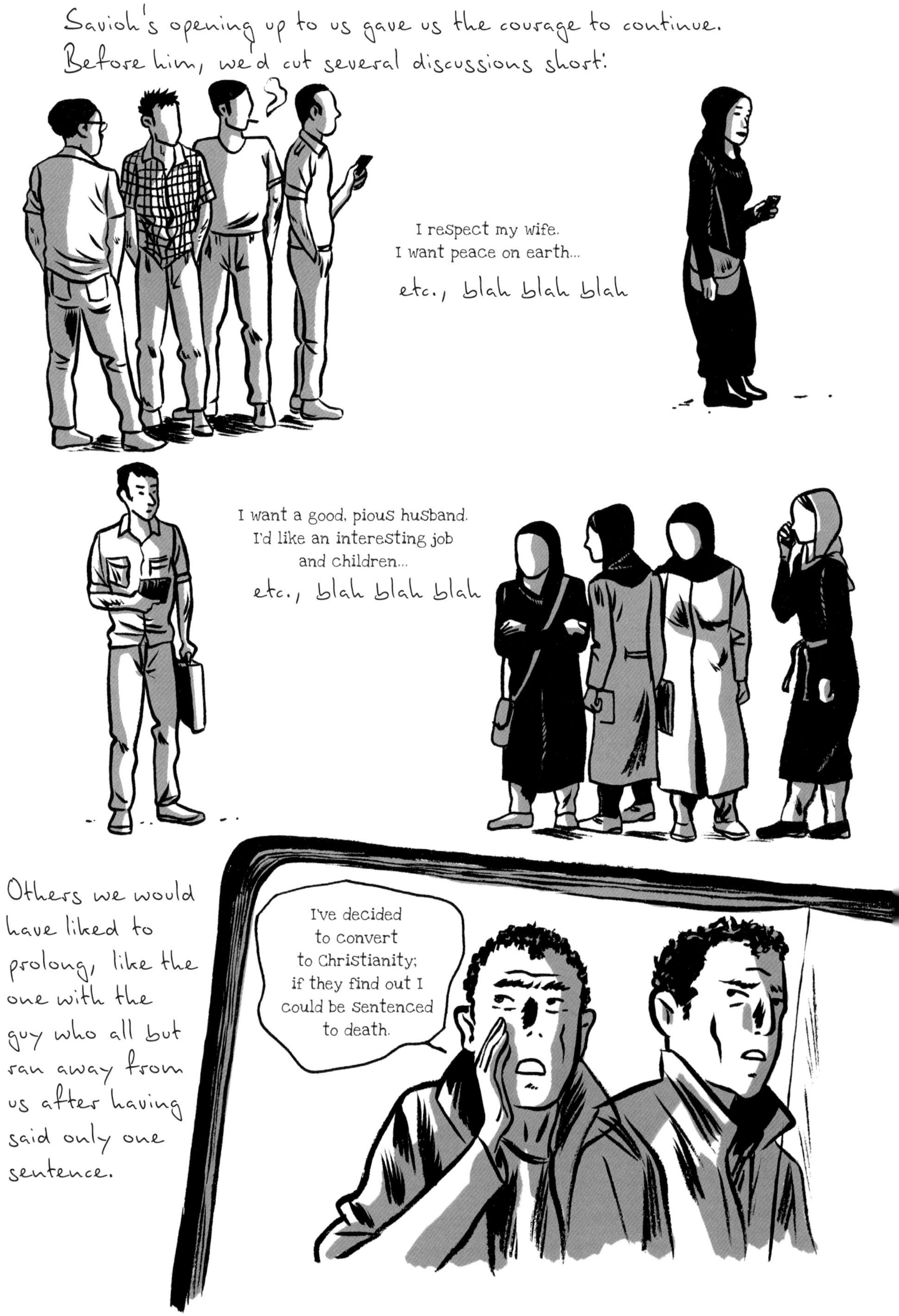
Savioh's opening up to us gave us the courage to continue. Before him, we'd cut several discussions short:
I respect my wife.
I want peace on earth...
etc., blah blah blah
I want a good, pious husband.
I'd like an interesting job
and children...
etc., blah blah blah
Others we would have liked to prolong, like the one with the guy who all but ran away from us after having said only one sentence.
I've decided to convert to Christianity; if they find out I could be sentenced to death.

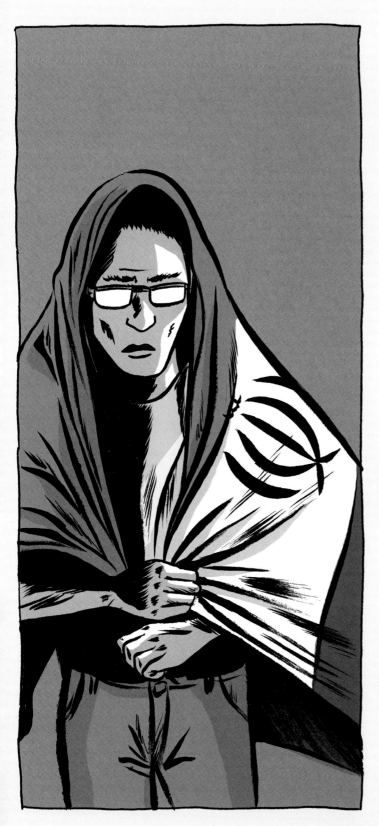

VAHID, 26,
Behesht-e
Zahra cemetery.

The biggest cemetery in Iran
is on the road to Kashan.
We met Vahid there.

He has nothing to lose and
wants to talk politics.

"Because I love my country."

My parents acted like
spoiled children.

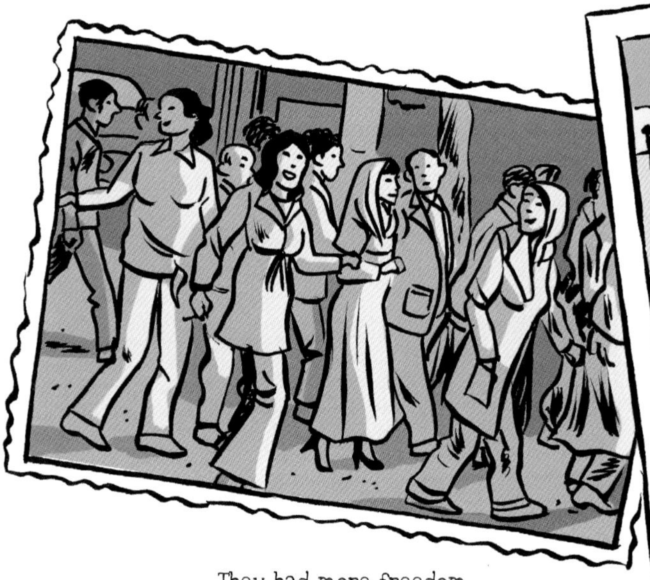

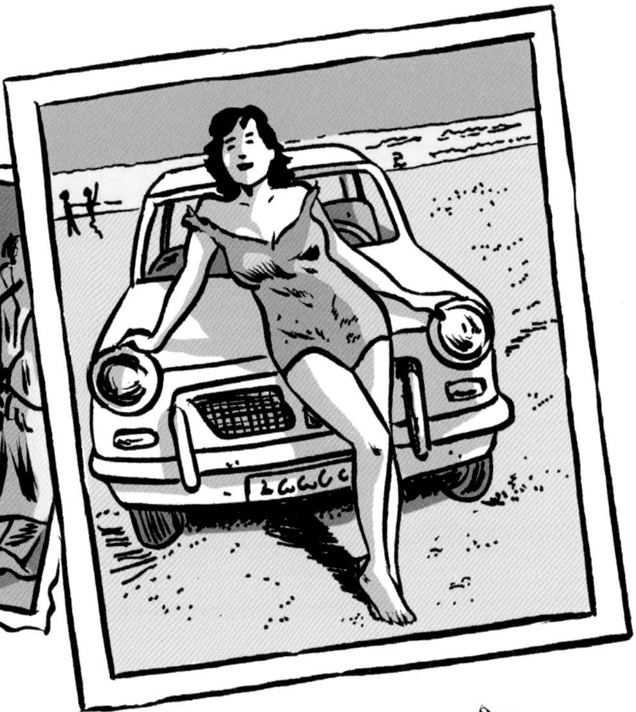

They had more freedom
than I'll ever have.

In 1979, they wanted a revolution, even
though the country was modernizing.

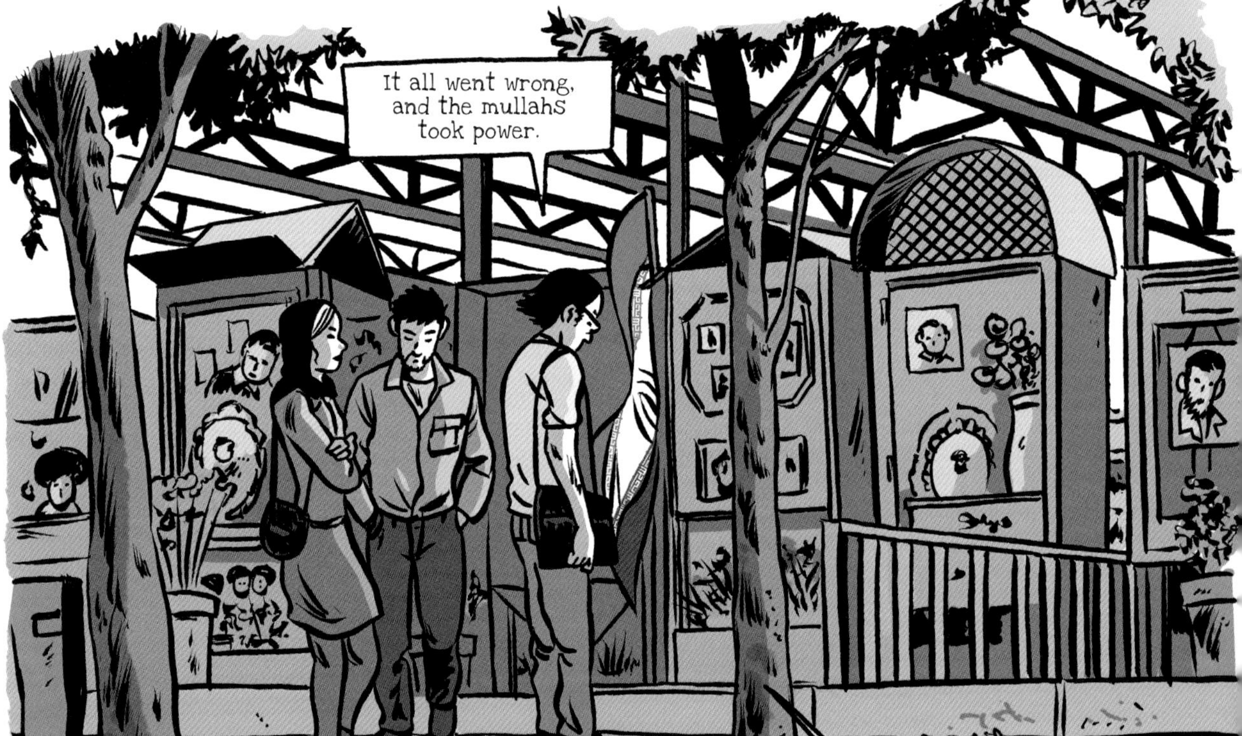
It all went wrong, and the mullahs took power.
And now I have to put up with the Islamic Republic.

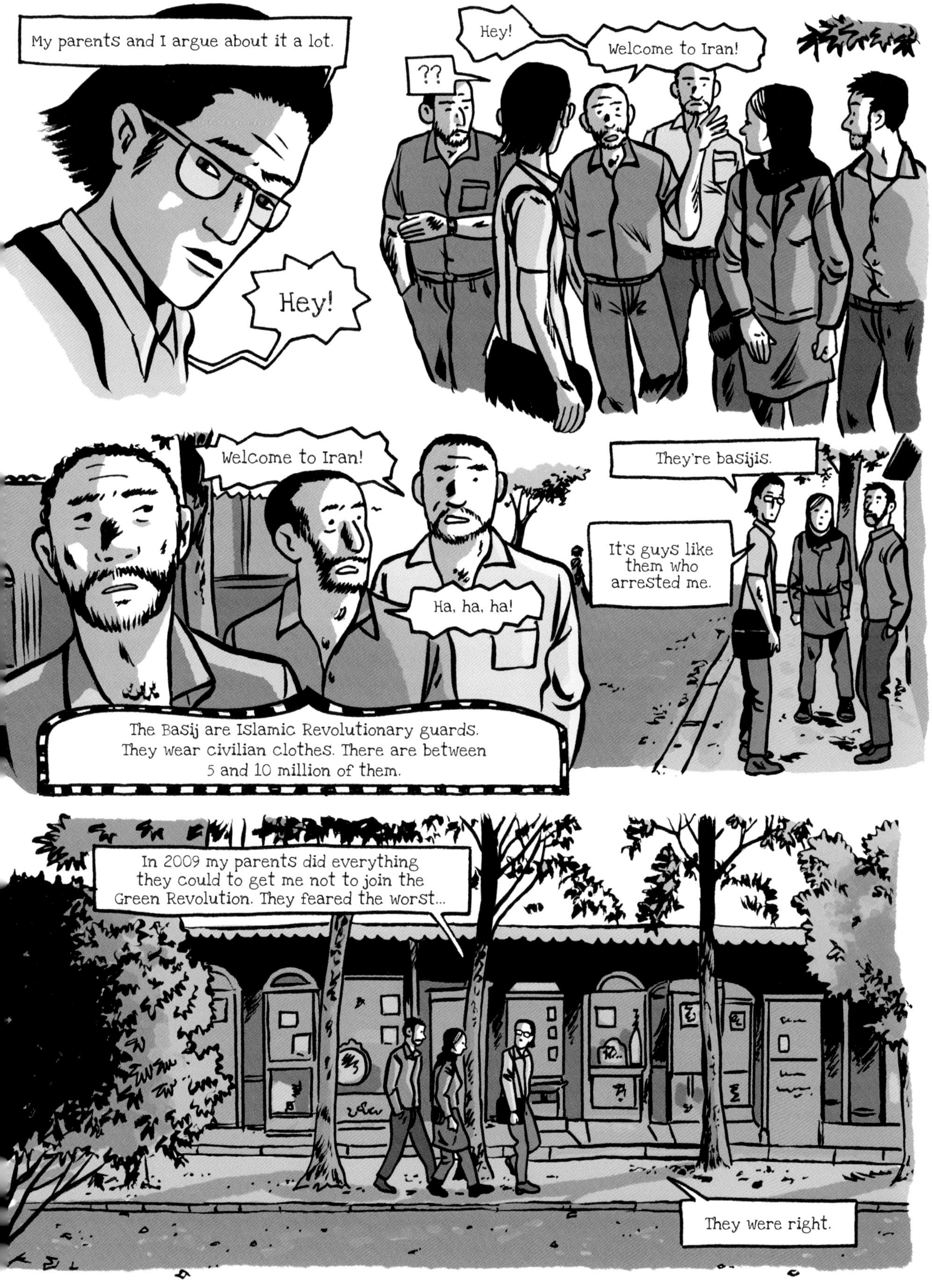
My parents and I argue about it a lot.
Hey!
Hey!
??
Welcome to Iran!
Welcome to Iran!
Ha, ha, ha!
The Basij are Islamic Revolutionary guards. They wear civilian clothes. There are between 5 and 10 million of them.
They're basijis.
It's guys like them who arrested me.
In 2009 my parents did everything they could to get me not to join the Green Revolution. They feared the worst...
They were right.

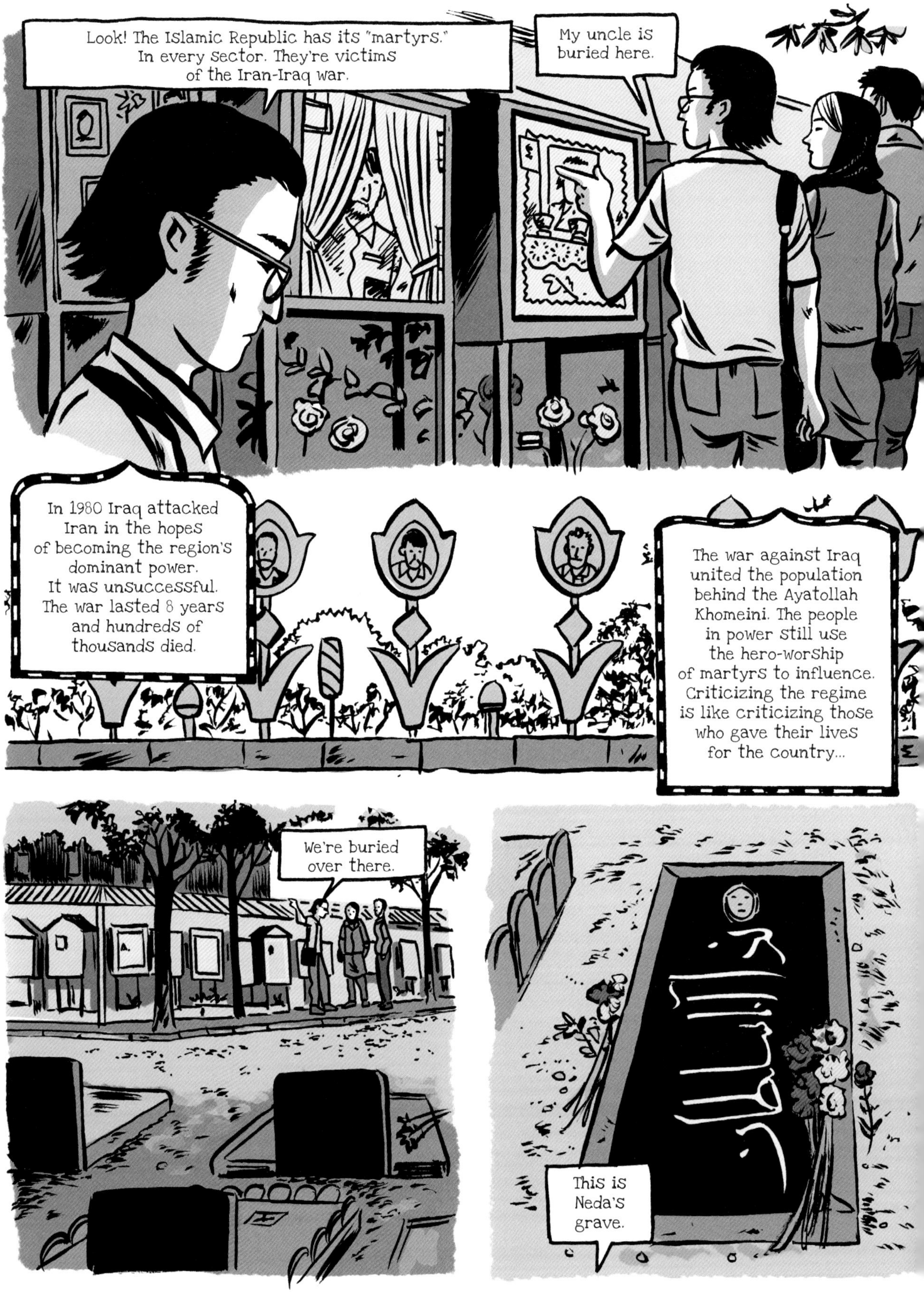
Look! The Islamic Republic has its "martyrs." In every sector. They're victims of the Iran-Iraq war.
My uncle is buried here.
In 1980 Iraq attacked Iran in the hopes of becoming the region's dominant power. It was unsuccessful. The war lasted 8 years and hundreds of thousands died.
The war against Iraq united the population behind the Ayatollah Khomeini. The people in power still use the hero-worship of martyrs to influence. Criticizing the regime is like criticizing those who gave their lives for the country...
We're buried over there.
This is Neda's grave.

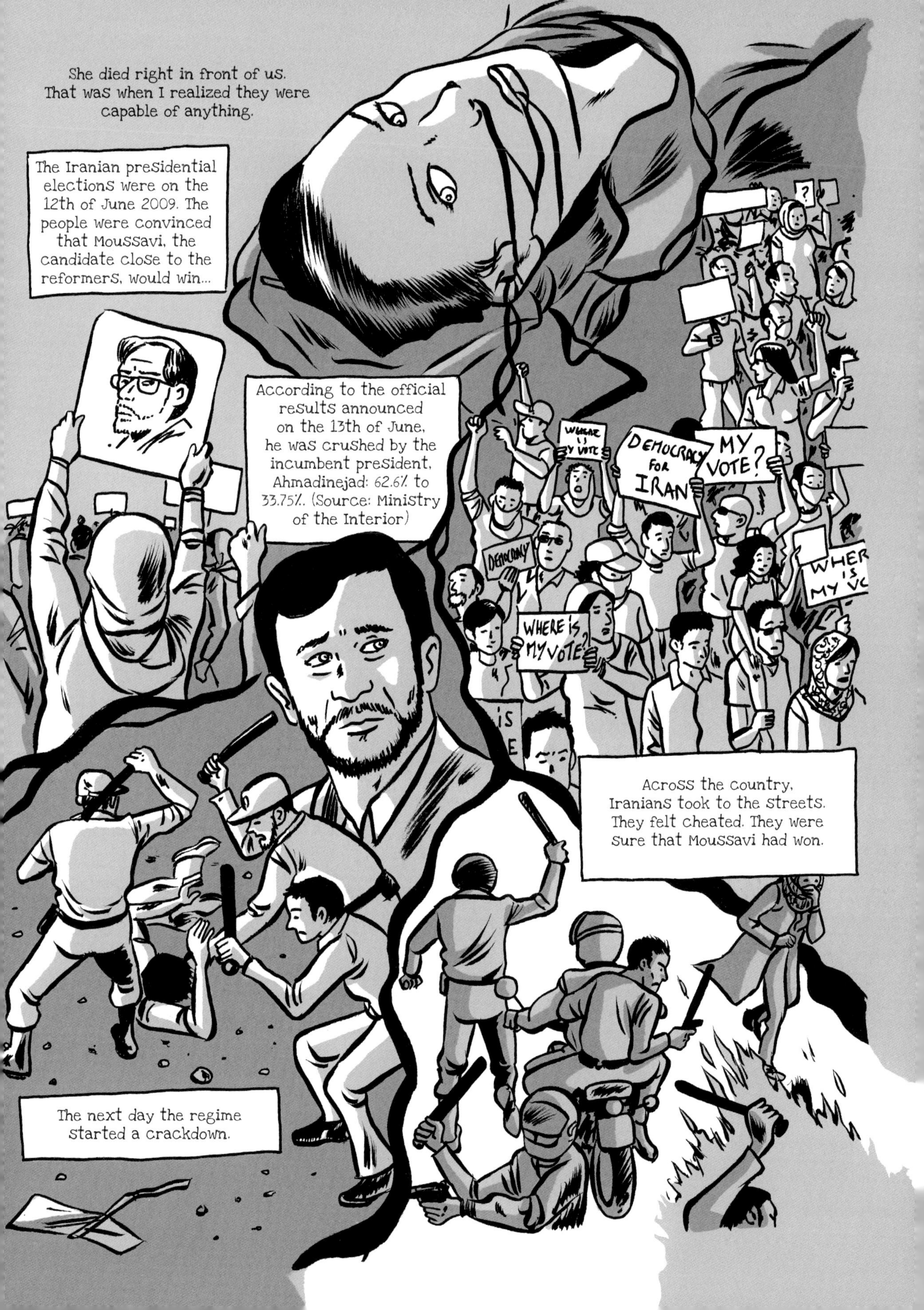
She died right in front of us. That was when I realized they were capable of anything.
The Iranian presidential elections were on the 12th of June 2009. The people were convinced that Moussavi, the candidate close to the reformers, would win...
According to the official results announced on the 13th of June, he was crushed by the incumbent president, Ahmadinejad: 62.6% to 33.75%. (Source: Ministry of the Interior)
DEMOCRACY FOR IRAN
MY VOTE?
DEMOCRACY
WHERE IS MY VOTE?
Across the country, Iranians took to the streets. They felt cheated. They were sure that Moussavi had won.
The next day the regime started a crackdown.

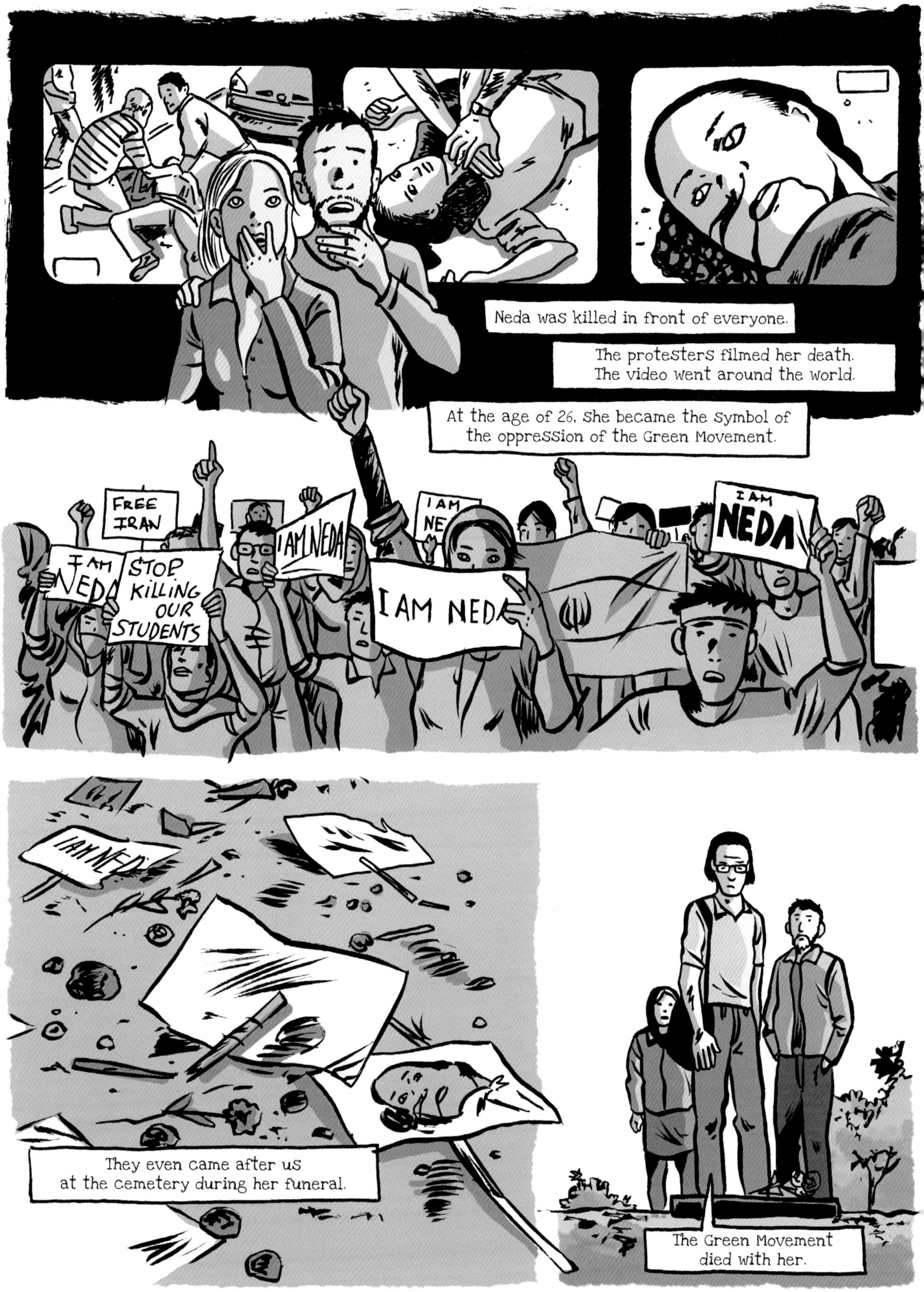
Neda was killed in front of everyone.
The protesters filmed her death. The video went around the world.
At the age of 26, she became the symbol of the oppression of the Green Movement.
FREE IRAN
I AM NEDA
STOP KILLING OUR STUDENTS
I AM NEDA
I AM NEDA
I AM NEDA
They even came after us at the cemetery during her funeral.
The Green Movement died with her.

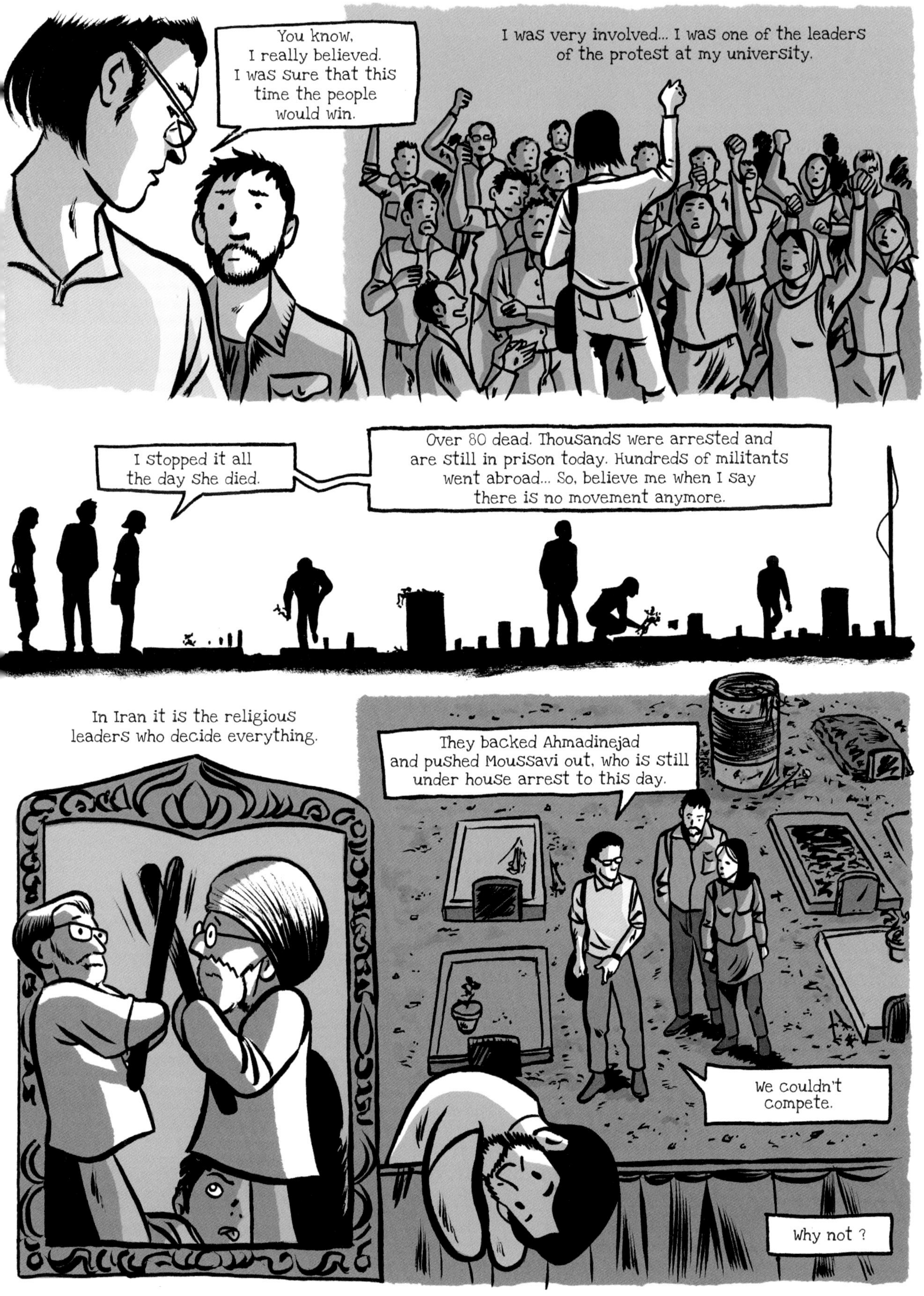
You know, I really believed. I was sure that this time the people would win.
I was very involved... I was one of the leaders of the protest at my university.
I stopped it all the day she died.
Over 80 dead. Thousands were arrested and are still in prison today. Hundreds of militants went abroad... So, believe me when I say there is no movement anymore.
In Iran it is the religious leaders who decide everything.
They backed Ahmadinejad and pushed Moussavi out, who is still under house arrest to this day.
We couldn't compete.
Why not ?

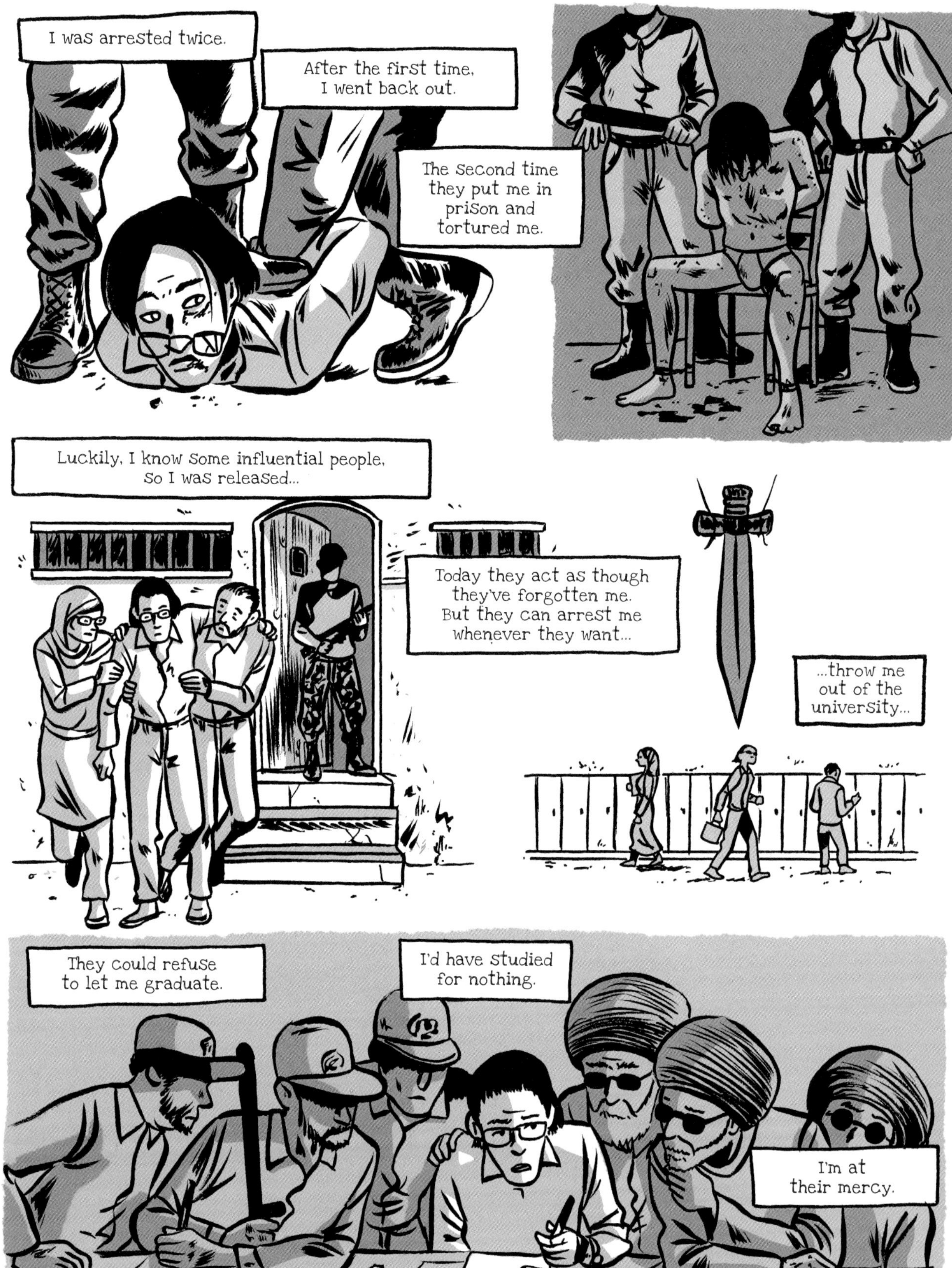

I was arrested twice.
After the first time, I went back out.
The second time they put me in prison and tortured me.
Luckily, I know some influential people, so I was released...
Today they act as though they've forgotten me. But they can arrest me whenever they want...
...throw me out of the university...
They could refuse to let me graduate.
I'd have studied for nothing.
I'm at their mercy.

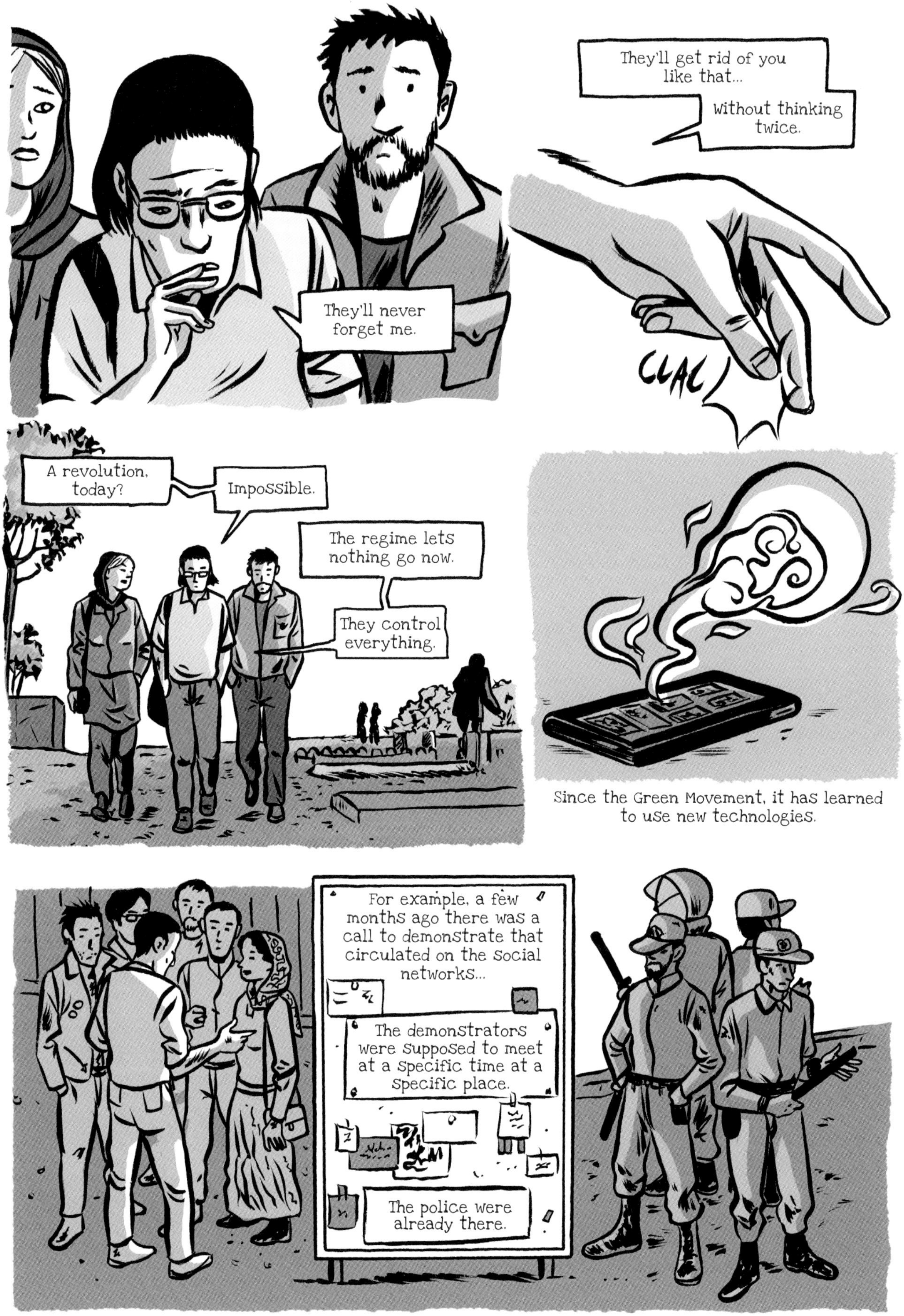
They'll never forget me.
They'll get rid of you like that...
Without thinking twice.
CLAC
A revolution, today?
Impossible.
The regime lets nothing go now.
They control everything.
Since the Green Movement, it has learned to use new technologies.
For example, a few months ago there was a call to demonstrate that circulated on the social networks...
The demonstrators were supposed to meet at a specific time at a specific place.
The police were already there.

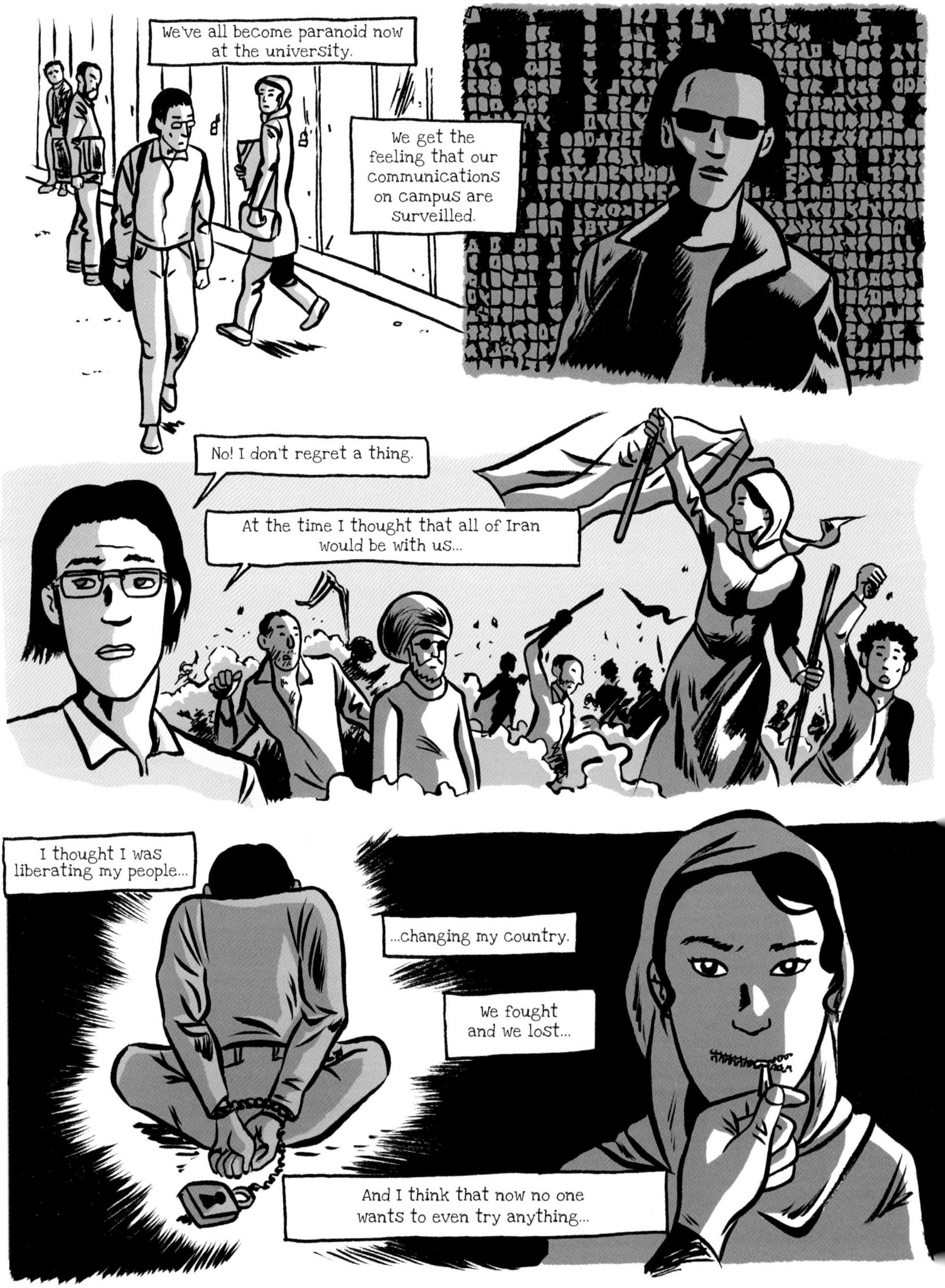
We've all become paranoid now at the university.
We get the feeling that our communications on campus are surveilled.
No! I don't regret a thing.
At the time I thought that all of Iran would be with us...
I thought I was liberating my people...
...changing my country.
We fought and we lost...
And I think that now no one wants to even try anything...

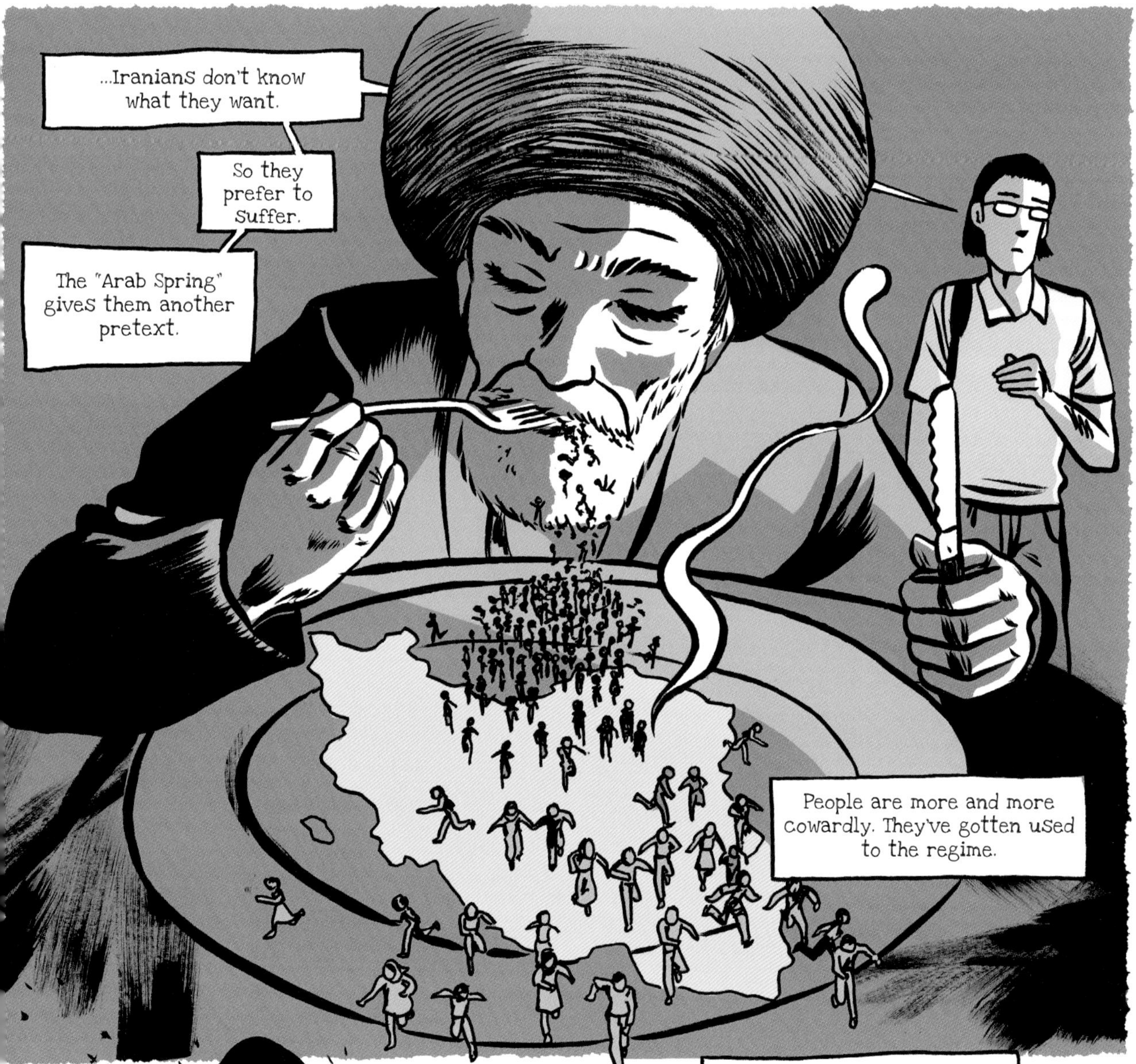
...Iranians don't know what they want.
So they prefer to suffer.
The "Arab Spring" gives them another pretext.
People are more and more cowardly. They've gotten used to the regime.

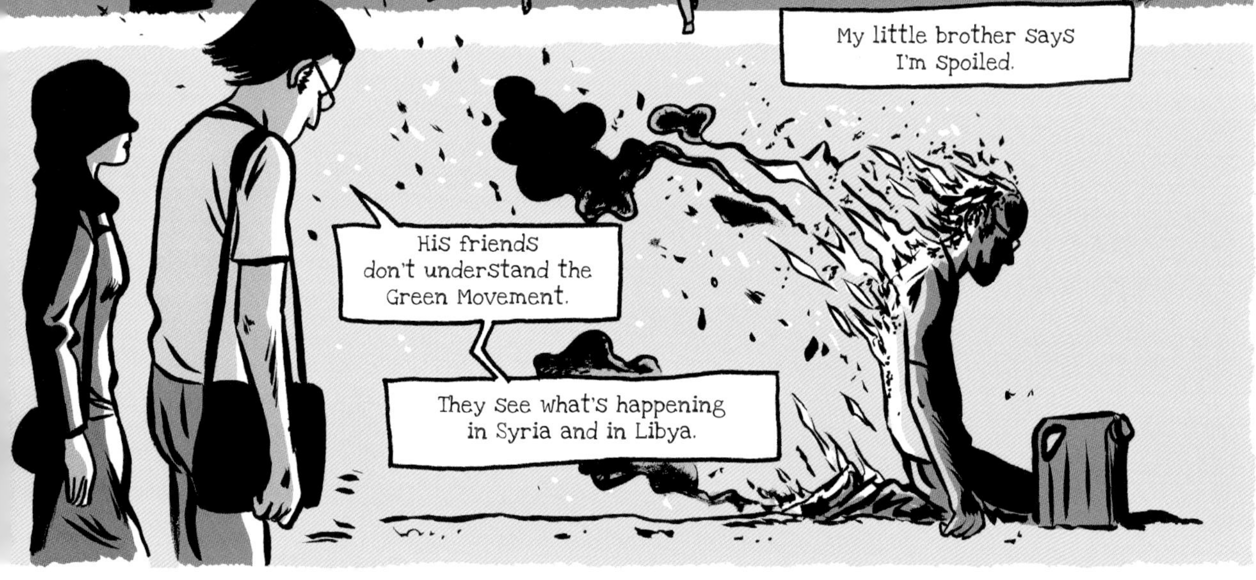
My little brother says I'm spoiled.
His friends don't understand the Green Movement.
They see what's happening in Syria and in Libya.

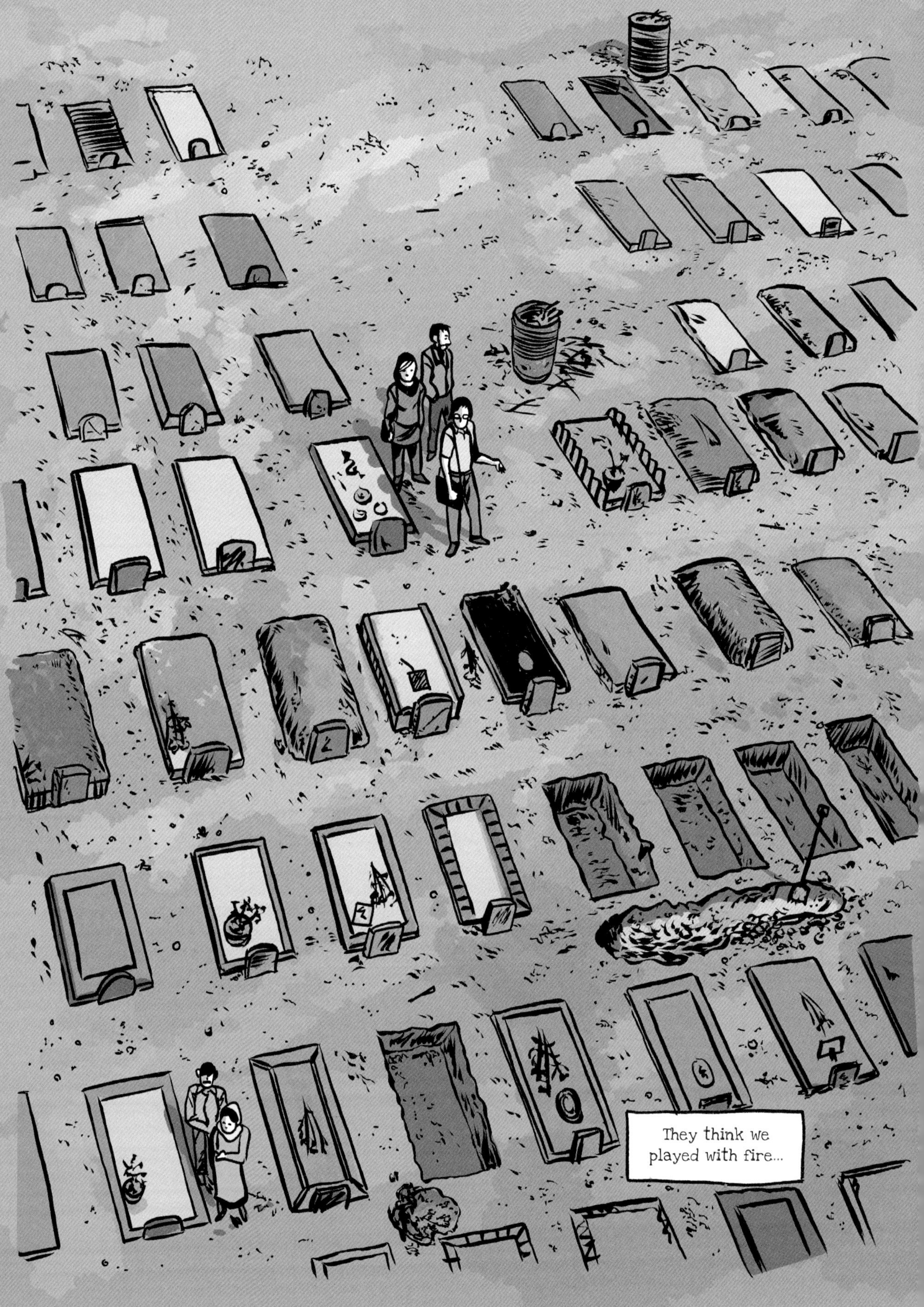
They think we played with fire...

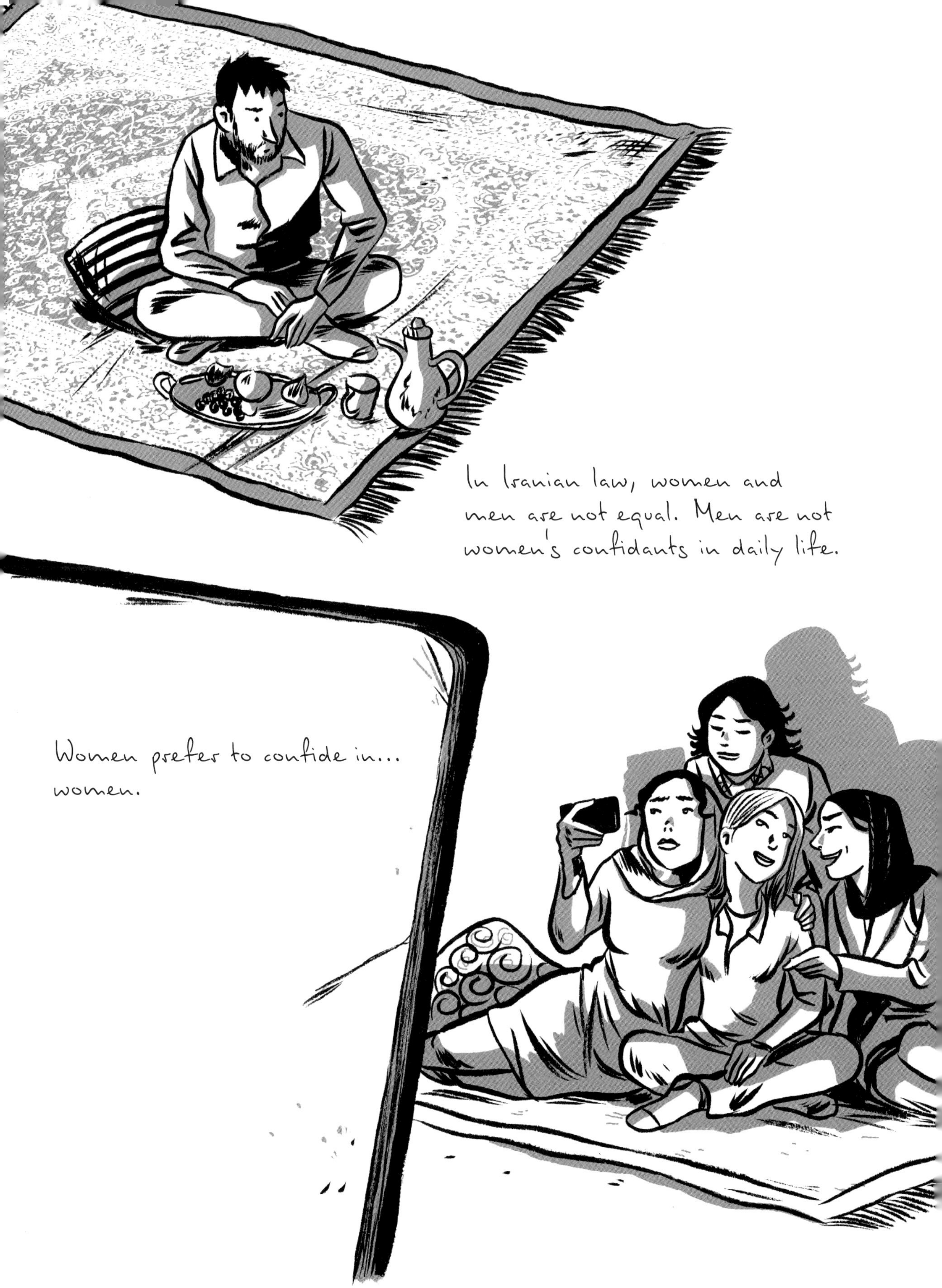
In Iranian law, women and men are not equal. Men are not women's confidants in daily life.
Women prefer to confide in... women.

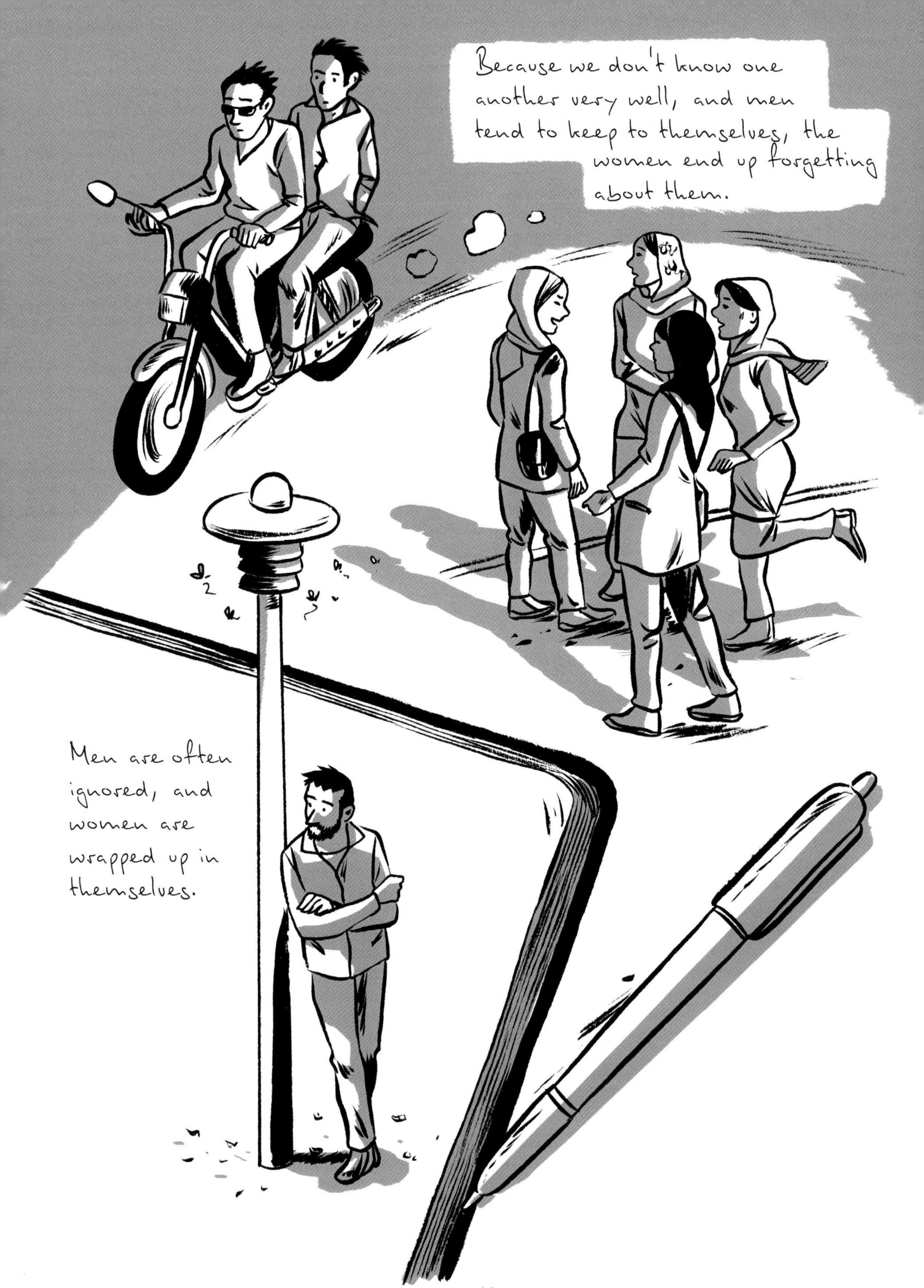
Because we don't know one another very well, and men tend to keep to themselves, the women end up forgetting about them.
Men are often ignored, and women are wrapped up in themselves.

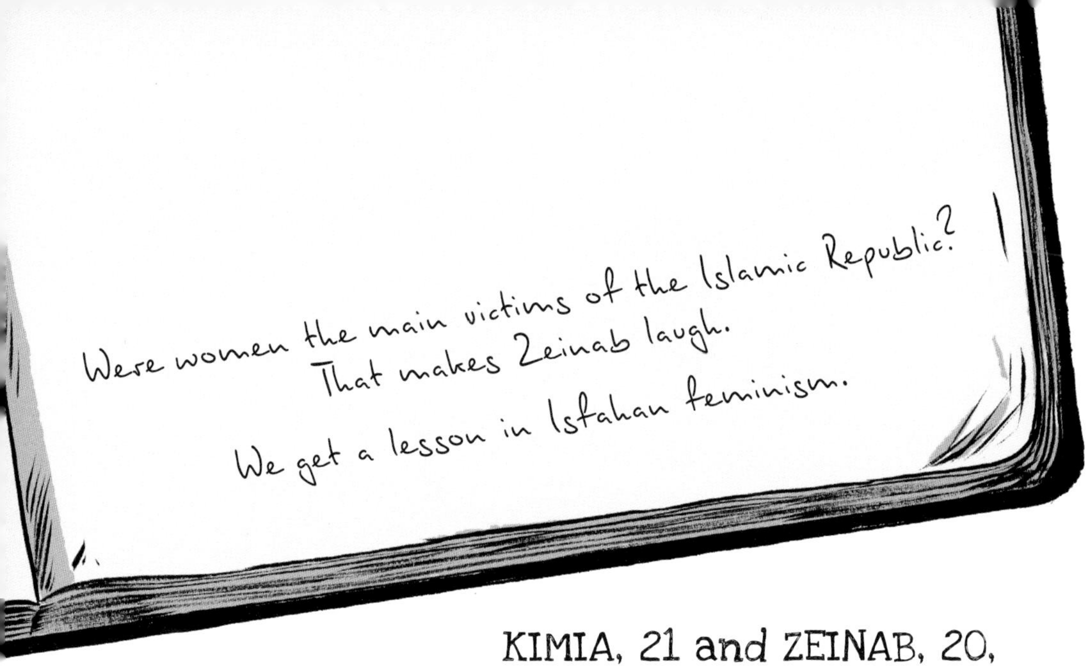
Were women the main victims of the Islamic Republic?
That makes Zeinab laugh.
We get a lesson in Isfahan feminism.

KIMIA, 21 and ZEINAB, 20,
Isfahan.

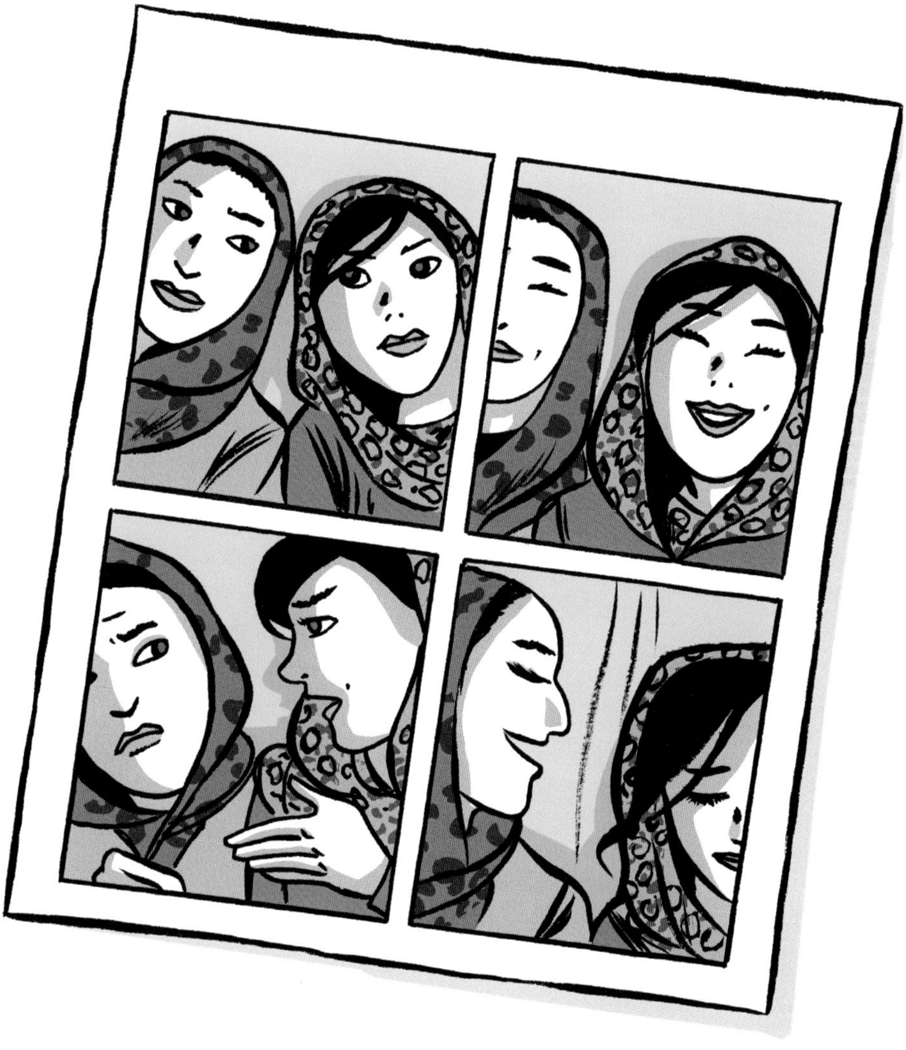

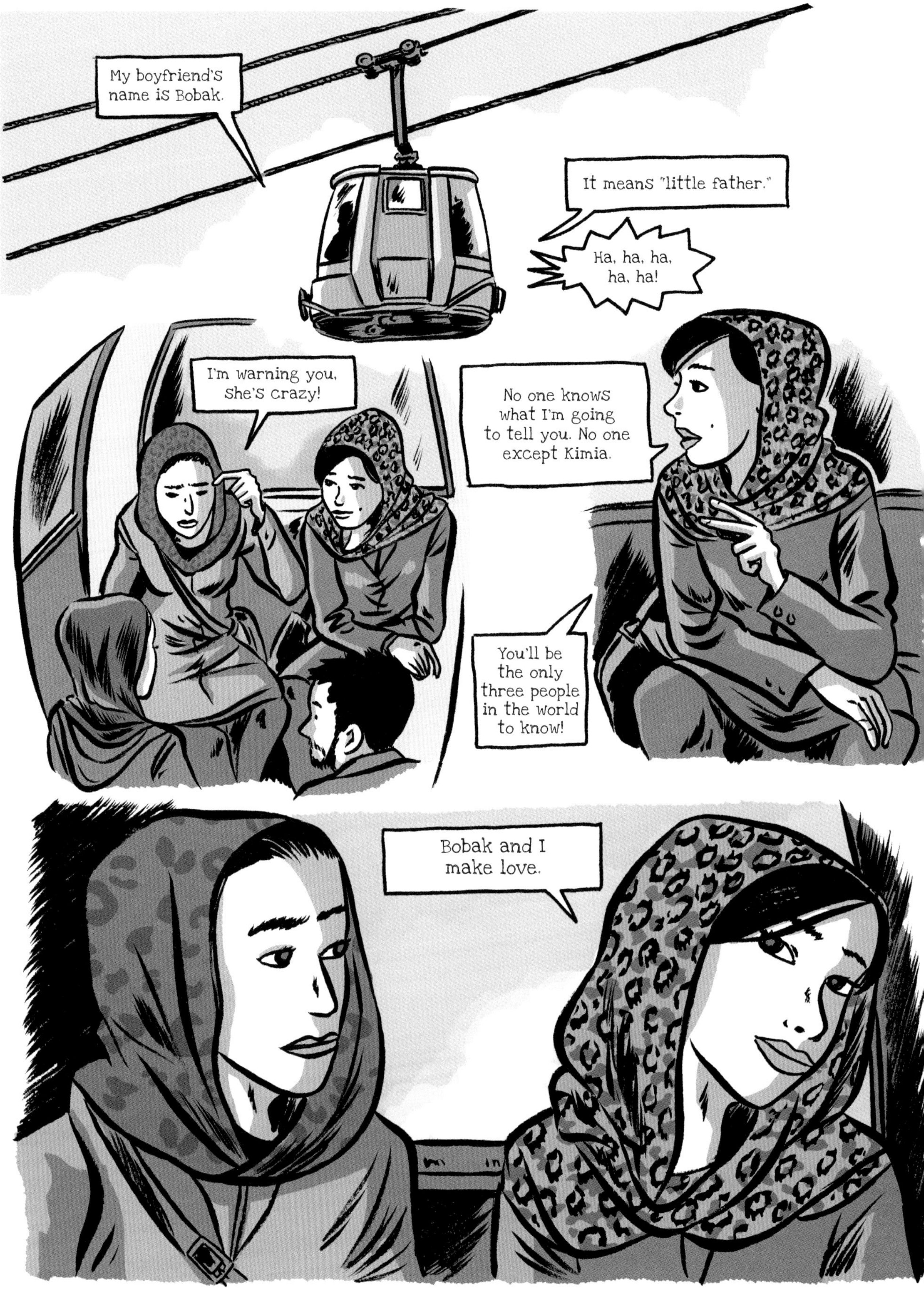
My boyfriend's name is Bobak.
It means "little father."
Ha, ha, ha, ha, ha!
I'm warning you, she's crazy!
No one knows what I'm going to tell you. No one except Kimia.
You'll be the only three people in the world to know!
Bobak and I make love.

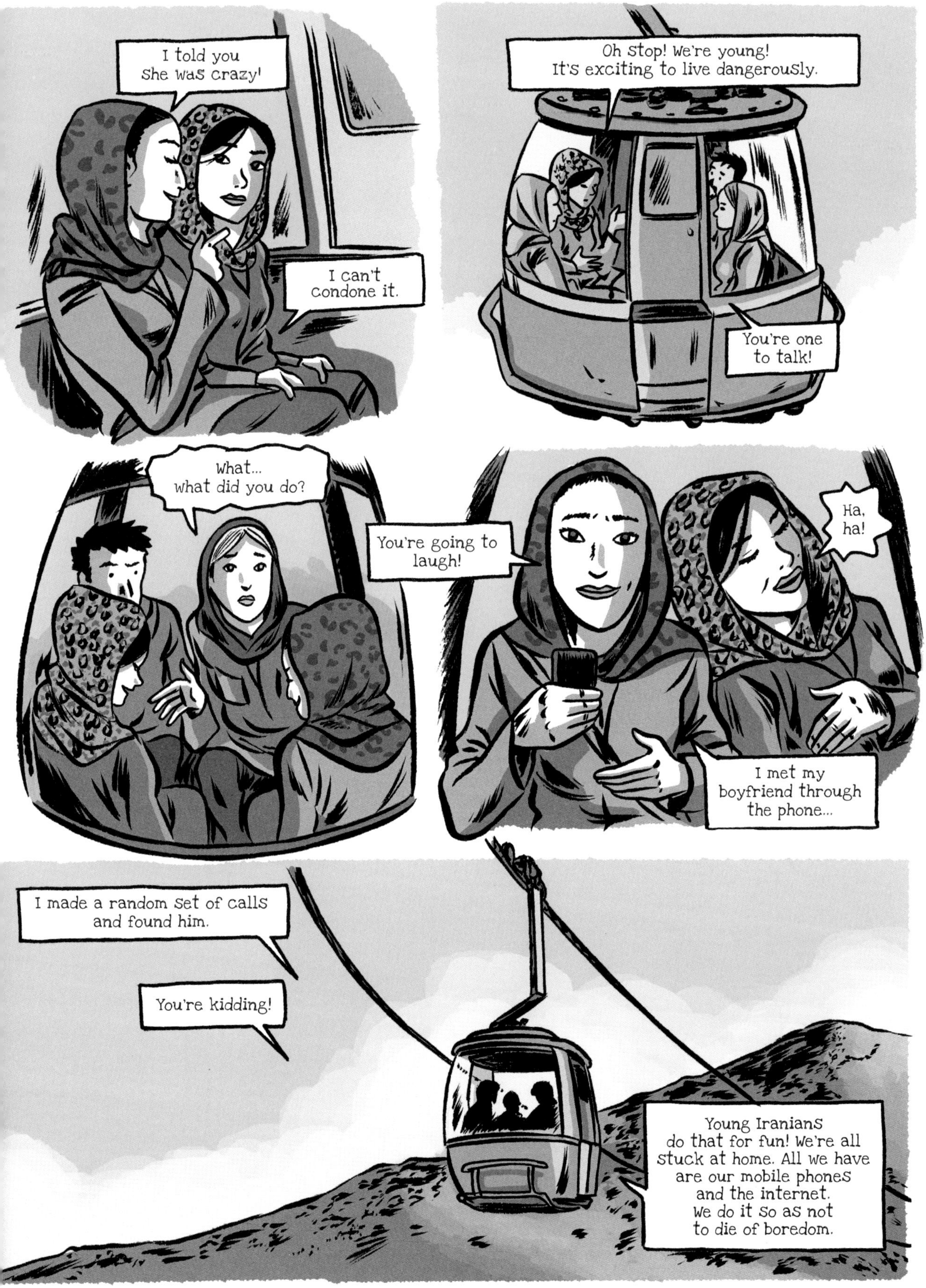
I told you she was crazy!
I can't condone it.
Oh stop! We're young! It's exciting to live dangerously.
You're one to talk!
What... what did you do?
You're going to laugh!
Ha, ha!
I met my boyfriend through the phone...
I made a random set of calls and found him.
You're kidding!
Young Iranians do that for fun! We're all stuck at home. All we have are our mobile phones and the internet. We do it so as not to die of boredom.

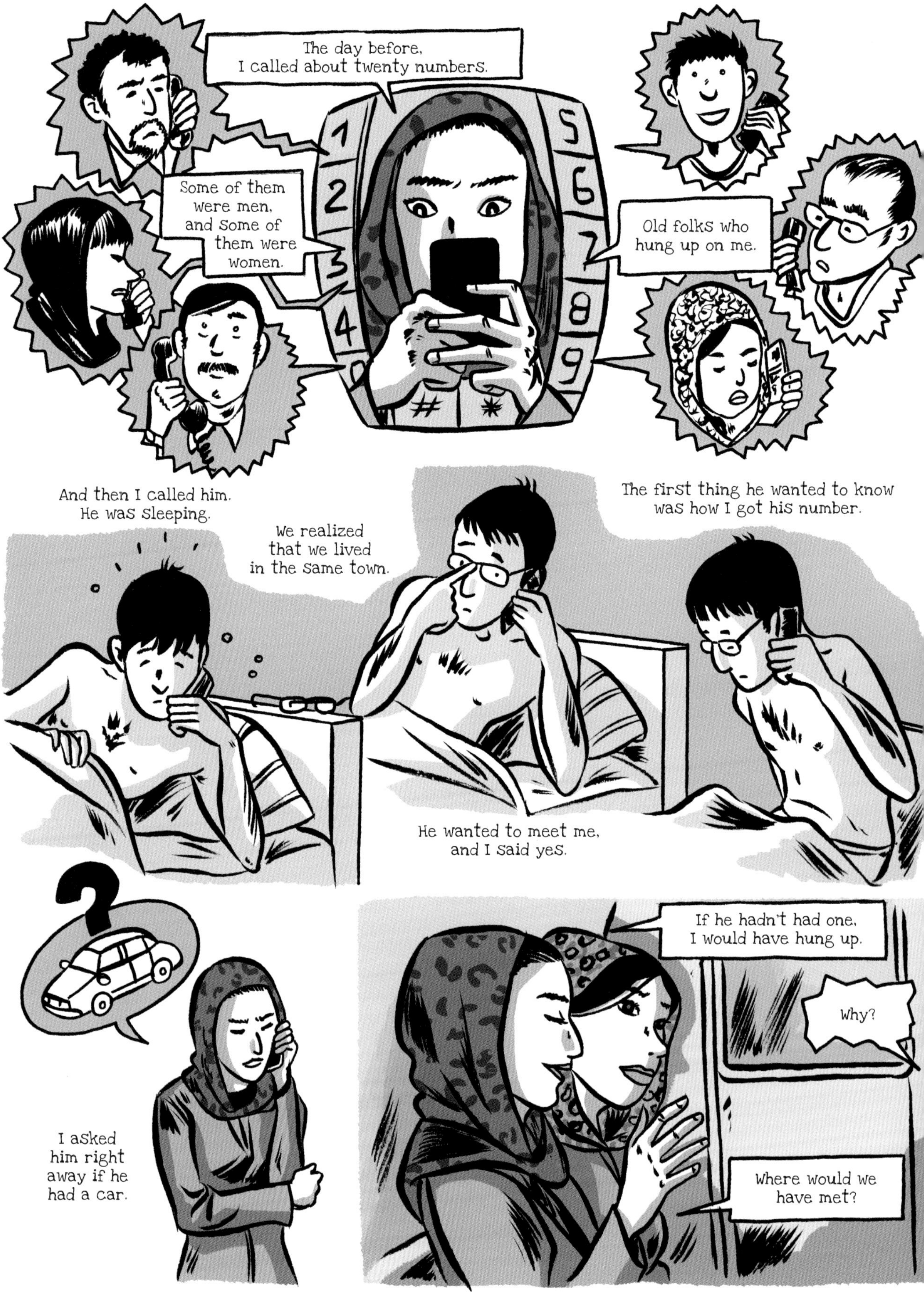
The day before, I called about twenty numbers.
Some of them were men, and some of them were women.
Old folks who hung up on me.
And then I called him. He was sleeping.
We realized that we lived in the same town.
The first thing he wanted to know was how I got his number.
He wanted to meet me, and I said yes.
I asked him right away if he had a car.
If he hadn't had one, I would have hung up.
Why?
Where would we have met?

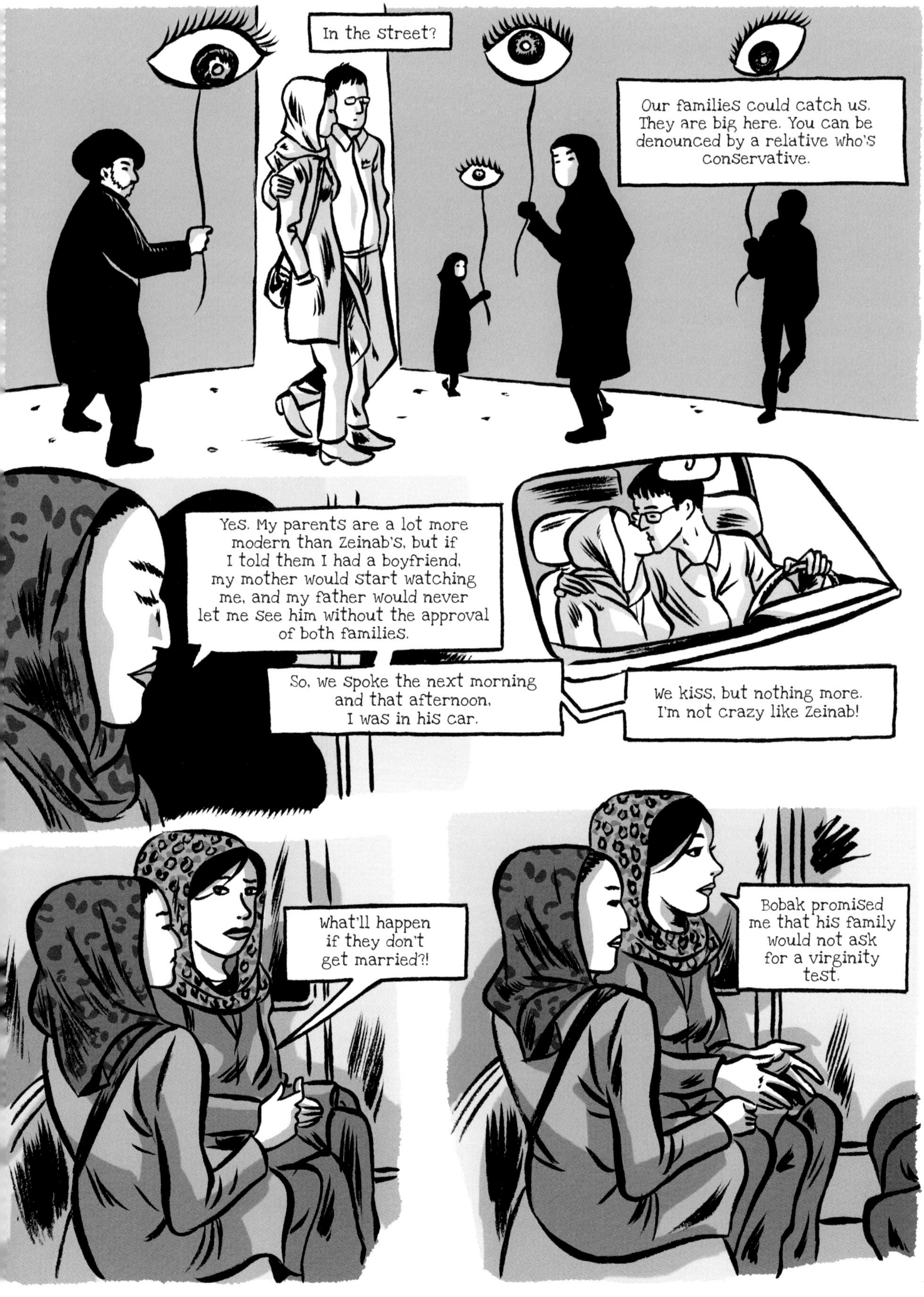
In the street?
Our families could catch us. They are big here. You can be denounced by a relative who's conservative.
Yes. My parents are a lot more modern than Zeinab's, but if I told them I had a boyfriend, my mother would start watching me, and my father would never let me see him without the approval of both families.
So, we spoke the next morning and that afternoon, I was in his car.
We kiss, but nothing more. I'm not crazy like Zeinab!
What'll happen if they don't get married?!
Bobak promised me that his family would not ask for a virginity test.

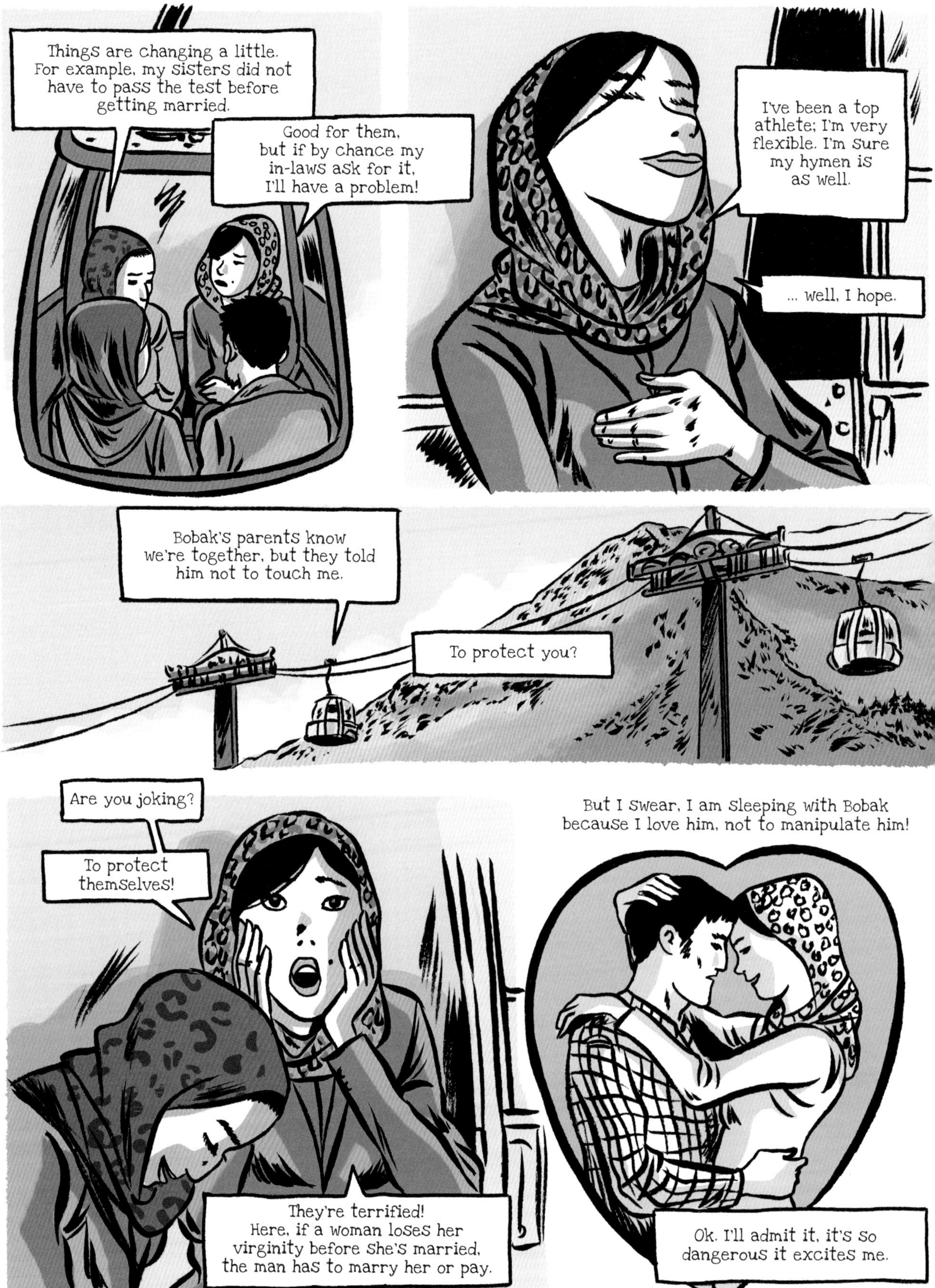
Things are changing a little. For example, my sisters did not have to pass the test before getting married.
Good for them, but if by chance my in-laws ask for it, I'll have a problem!
I've been a top athlete; I'm very flexible. I'm sure my hymen is as well.
... well, I hope.
Bobak's parents know we're together, but they told him not to touch me.
To protect you?
Are you joking?
To protect themselves!
They're terrified! Here, if a woman loses her virginity before she's married, the man has to marry her or pay.
But I swear, I am sleeping with Bobak because I love him, not to manipulate him!
Ok. I'll admit it, it's so dangerous it excites me.

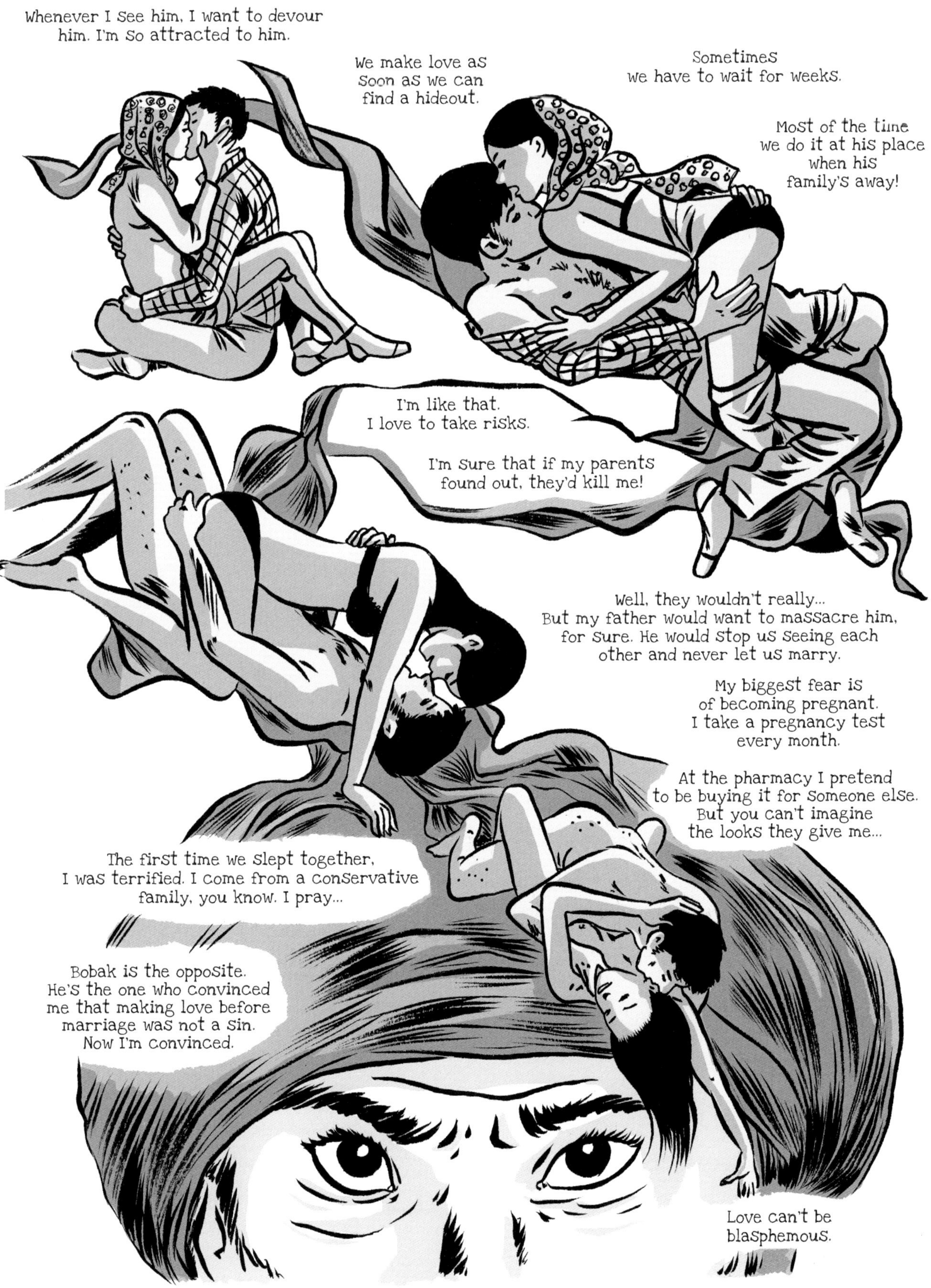
Whenever I see him, I want to devour him. I'm so attracted to him.
We make love as soon as we can find a hideout.
Sometimes we have to wait for weeks.
Most of the time we do it at his place when his family's away!
I'm like that. I love to take risks.
I'm sure that if my parents found out, they'd kill me!
Well, they wouldn't really... But my father would want to massacre him, for sure. He would stop us seeing each other and never let us marry.
My biggest fear is of becoming pregnant. I take a pregnancy test every month.
At the pharmacy I pretend to be buying it for someone else. But you can't imagine the looks they give me...
The first time we slept together, I was terrified. I come from a conservative family, you know. I pray...
Bobak is the opposite. He's the one who convinced me that making love before marriage was not a sin. Now I'm convinced.
Love can't be blasphemous.

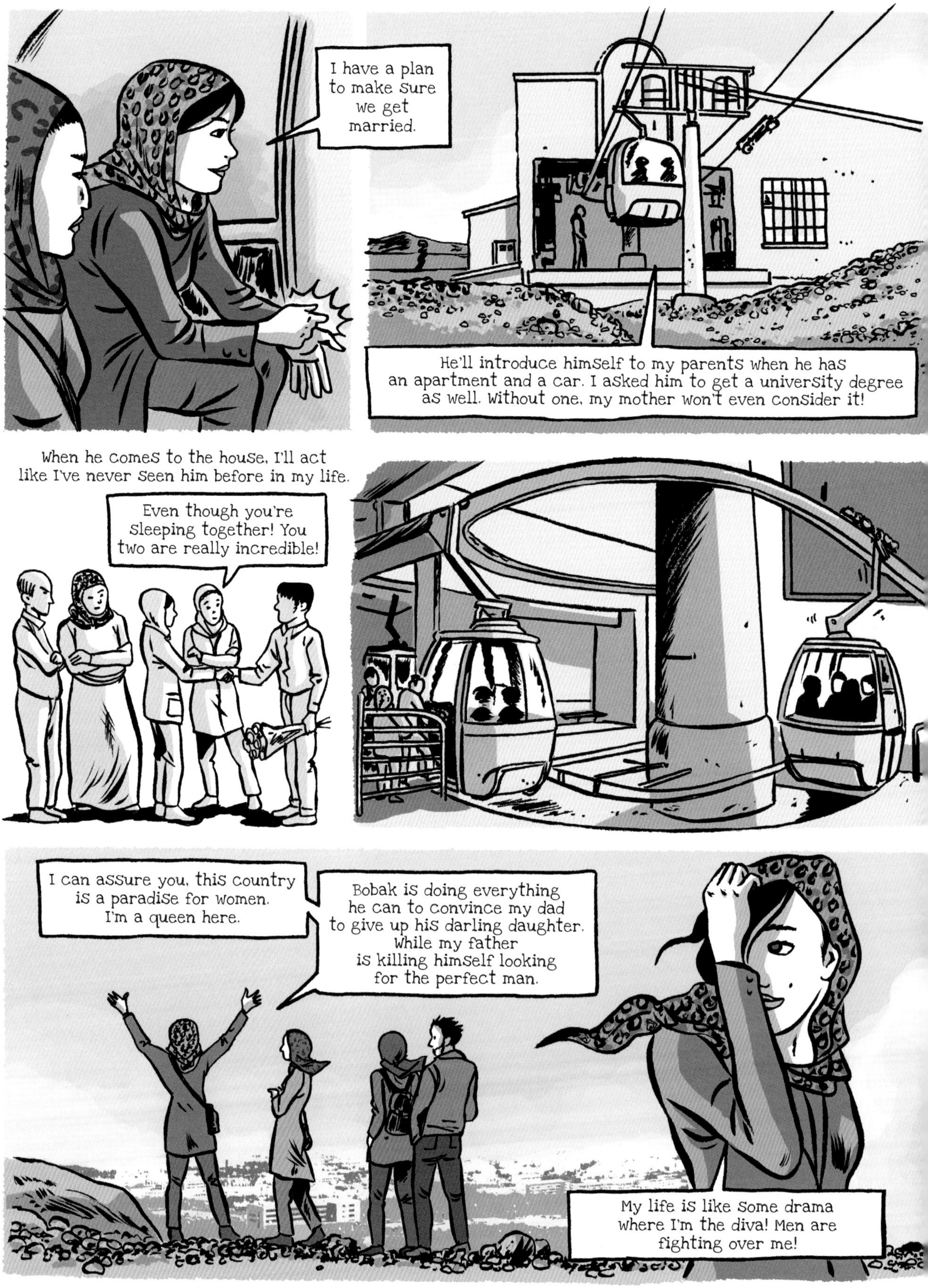

I have a plan to make sure we get married.
He'll introduce himself to my parents when he has an apartment and a car. I asked him to get a university degree as well. Without one, my mother won't even consider it!
When he comes to the house, I'll act like I've never seen him before in my life.
Even though you're sleeping together! You two are really incredible!
I can assure you, this country is a paradise for women. I'm a queen here.
Bobak is doing everything he can to convince my dad to give up his darling daughter. While my father is killing himself looking for the perfect man.
My life is like some drama where I'm the diva! Men are fighting over me!

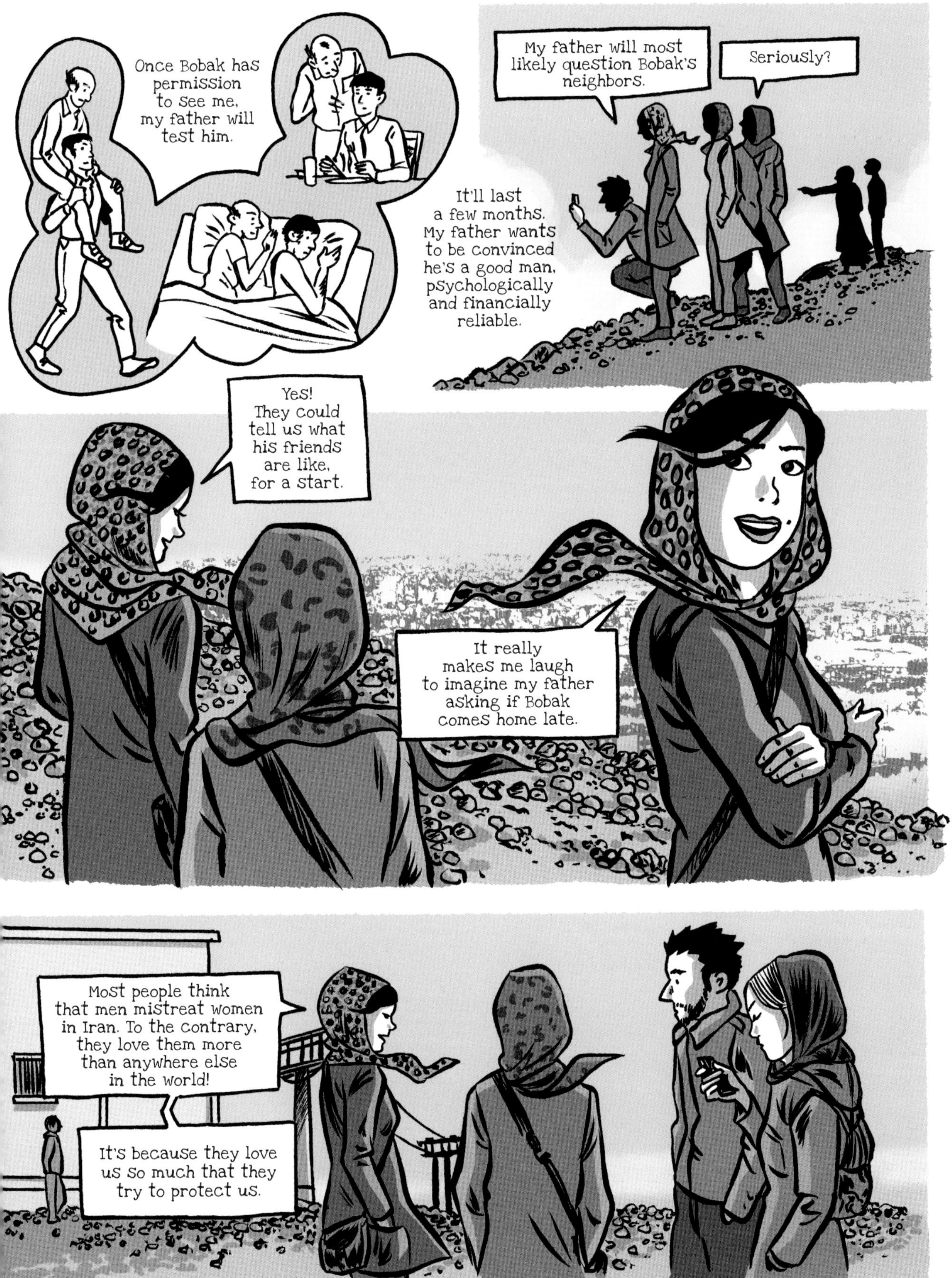
Once Bobak has permission to see me, my father will test him.
It'll last a few months. My father wants to be convinced he's a good man, psychologically and financially reliable.
My father will most likely question Bobak's neighbors.
Seriously?
Yes! They could tell us what his friends are like, for a start.
It really makes me laugh to imagine my father asking if Bobak comes home late.
Most people think that men mistreat women in Iran. To the contrary, they love them more than anywhere else in the world!
It's because they love us so much that they try to protect us.

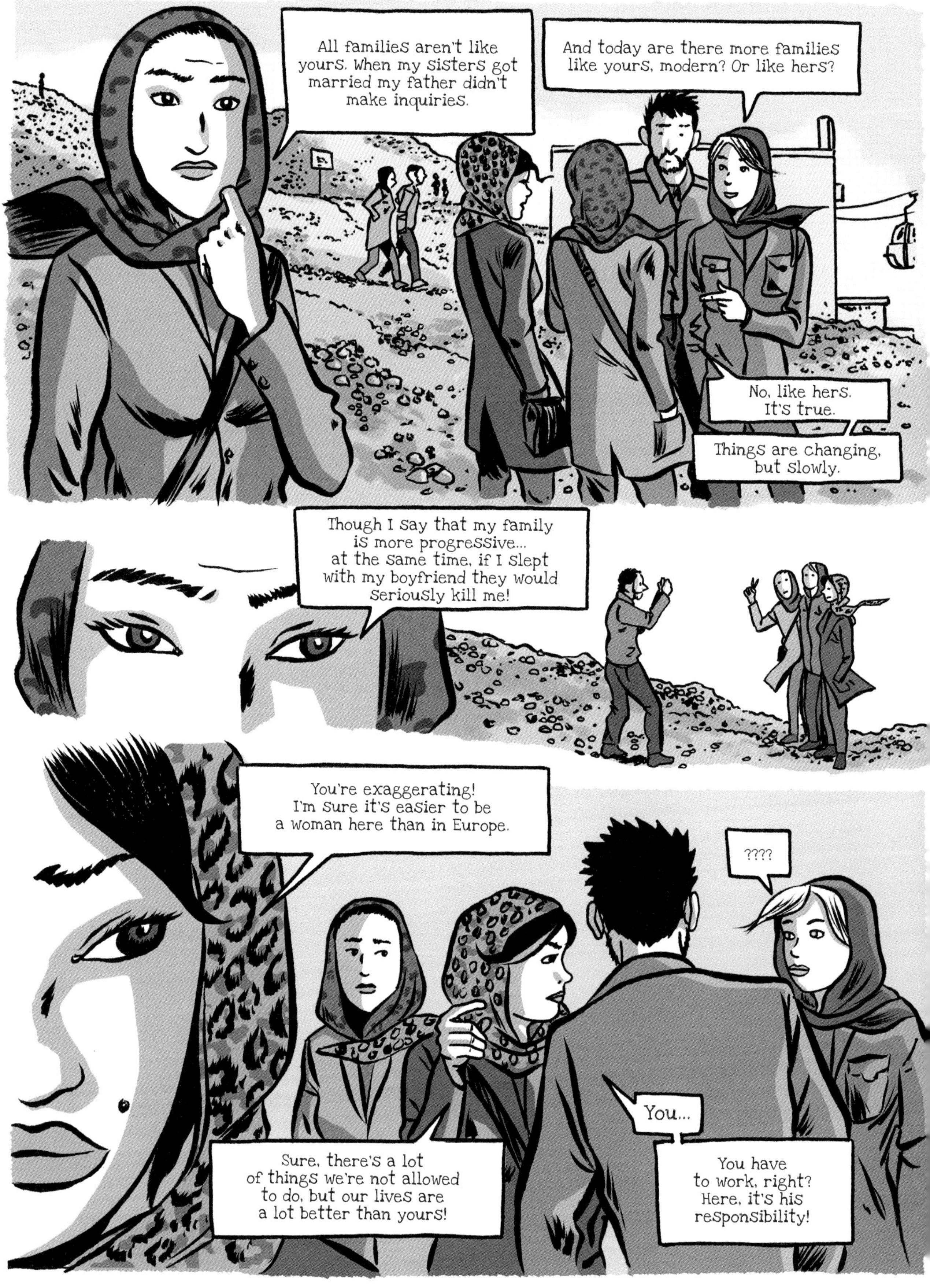
All families aren't like yours. When my sisters got married my father didn't make inquiries.
And today are there more families like yours, modern? Or like hers?
No, like hers. It's true.
Things are changing, but slowly.
Though I say that my family is more progressive... at the same time, if I slept with my boyfriend they would seriously kill me!
You're exaggerating! I'm sure it's easier to be a woman here than in Europe.
????
You...
Sure, there's a lot of things we're not allowed to do, but our lives are a lot better than yours!
You have to work, right? Here, it's his responsibility!

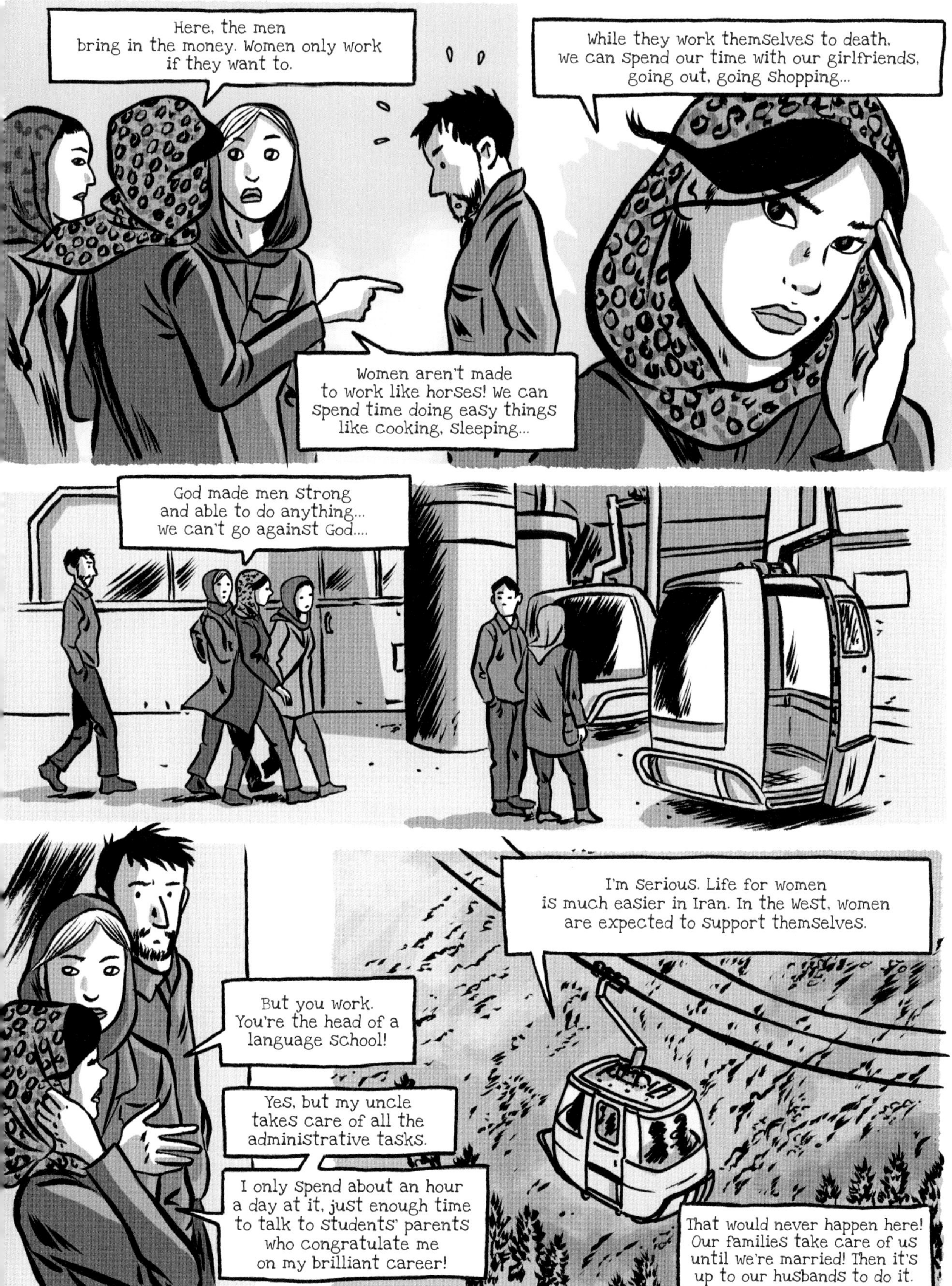
Here, the men bring in the money. Women only work if they want to.
While they work themselves to death, we can spend our time with our girlfriends, going out, going shopping...
Women aren't made to work like horses! We can spend time doing easy things like cooking, sleeping...
God made men strong and able to do anything... we can't go against God....
I'm serious. Life for women is much easier in Iran. In the West, women are expected to support themselves.
But you work. You're the head of a language school!
Yes, but my uncle takes care of all the administrative tasks.
I only spend about an hour a day at it, just enough time to talk to students' parents who congratulate me on my brilliant career!
That would never happen here! Our families take care of us until we're married! Then it's up to our husbands to do it.

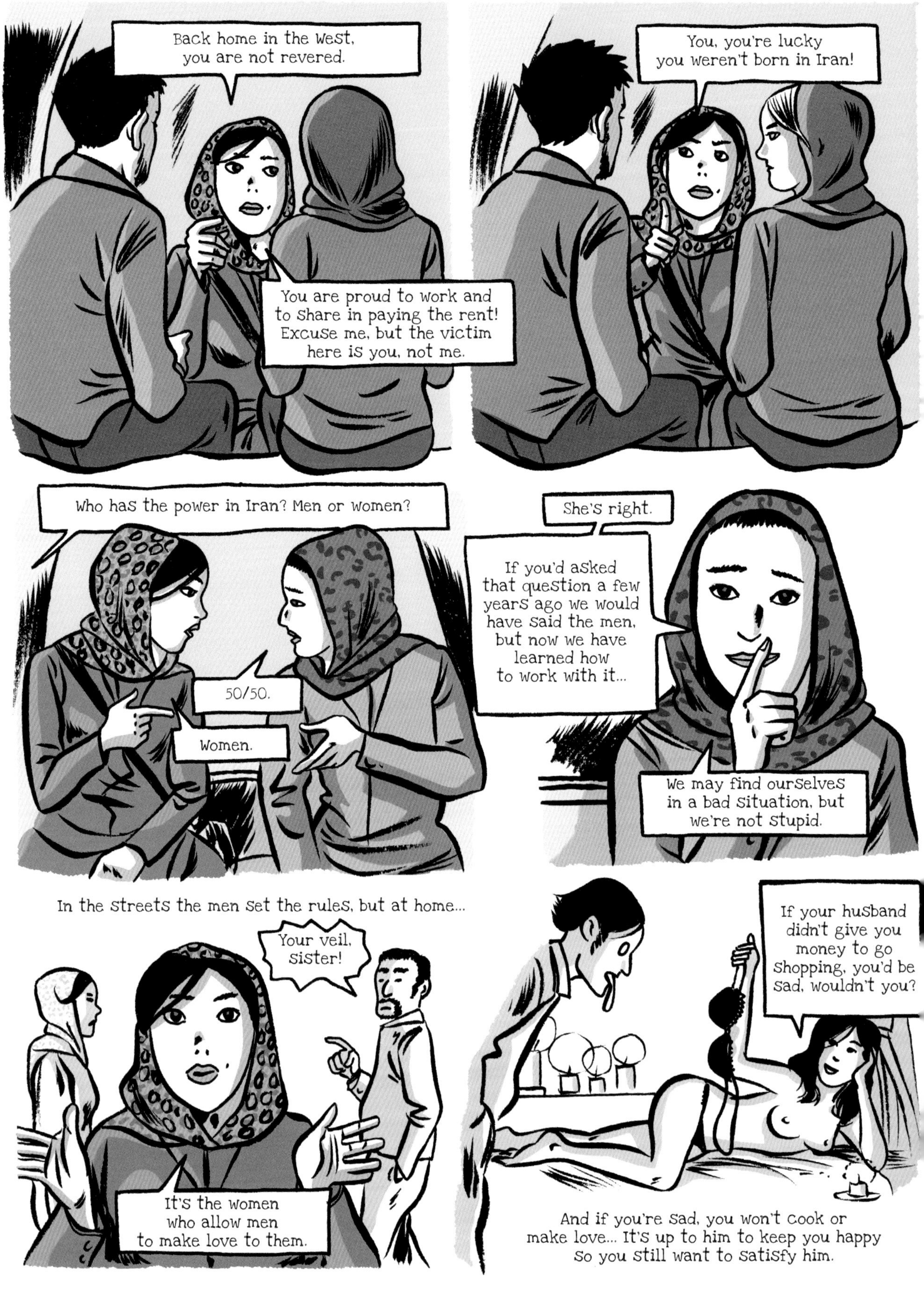
Back home in the West, you are not revered.
You are proud to work and to share in paying the rent! Excuse me, but the victim here is you, not me.
You, you're lucky you weren't born in Iran!
Who has the power in Iran? Men or women?
50/50.
Women.
She's right.
If you'd asked that question a few years ago we would have said the men, but now we have learned how to work with it...
We may find ourselves in a bad situation, but we're not stupid.
In the streets the men set the rules, but at home...
Your veil, sister!
It's the women who allow men to make love to them.
If your husband didn't give you money to go shopping, you'd be sad, wouldn't you?
And if you're sad, you won't cook or make love... It's up to him to keep you happy so you still want to satisfy him.

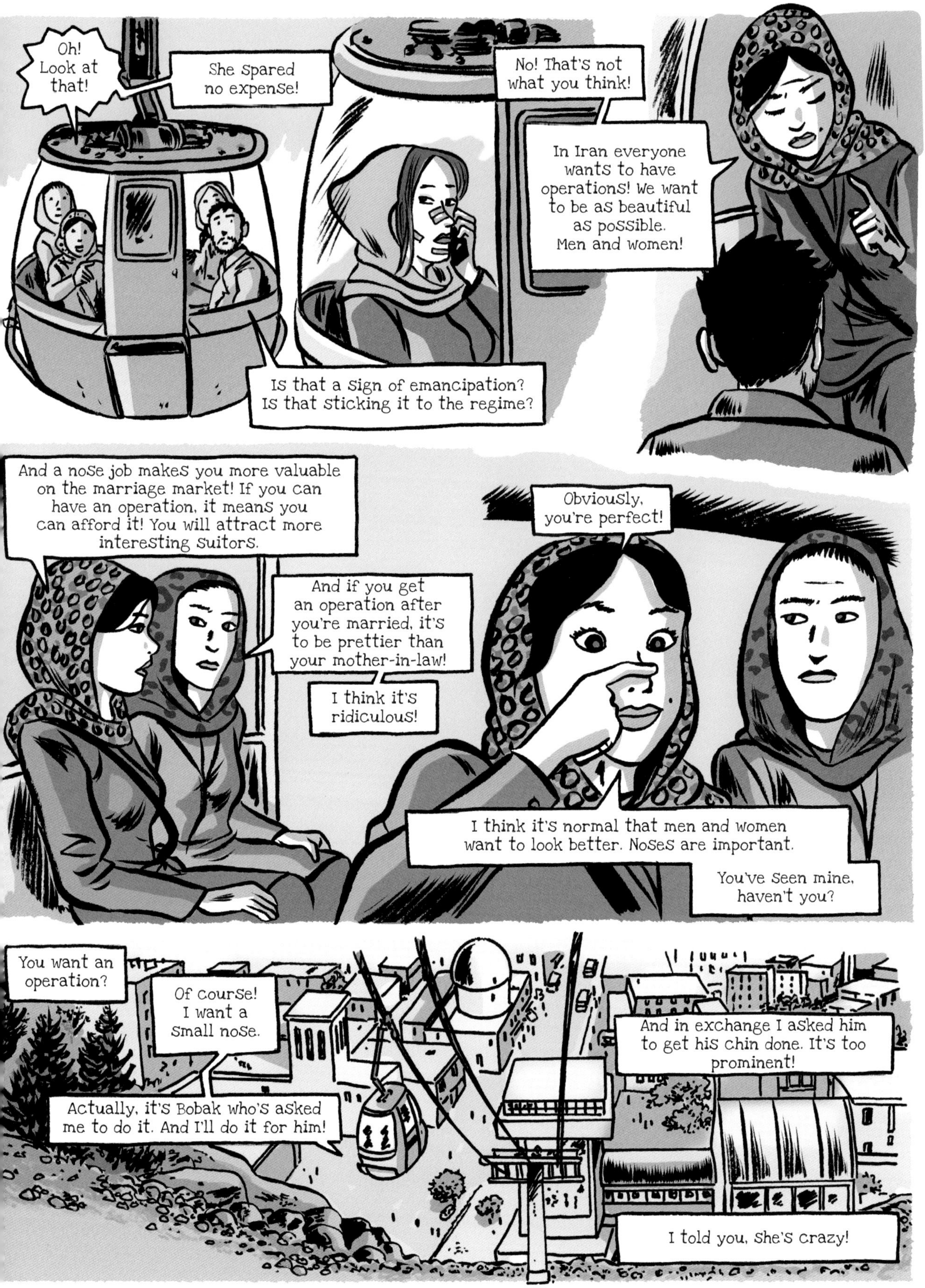

Oh! Look at that!
She spared no expense!
Is that a sign of emancipation? Is that sticking it to the regime?
No! That's not what you think!
In Iran everyone wants to have operations! We want to be as beautiful as possible. Men and women!
And a nose job makes you more valuable on the marriage market! If you can have an operation, it means you can afford it! You will attract more interesting suitors.
And if you get an operation after you're married, it's to be prettier than your mother-in-law!
I think it's ridiculous!
Obviously, you're perfect!
I think it's normal that men and women want to look better. Noses are important.
You've seen mine, haven't you?
You want an operation?
Of course! I want a small nose.
Actually, it's Bobak who's asked me to do it. And I'll do it for him!
And in exchange I asked him to get his chin done. It's too prominent!
I told you, she's crazy!

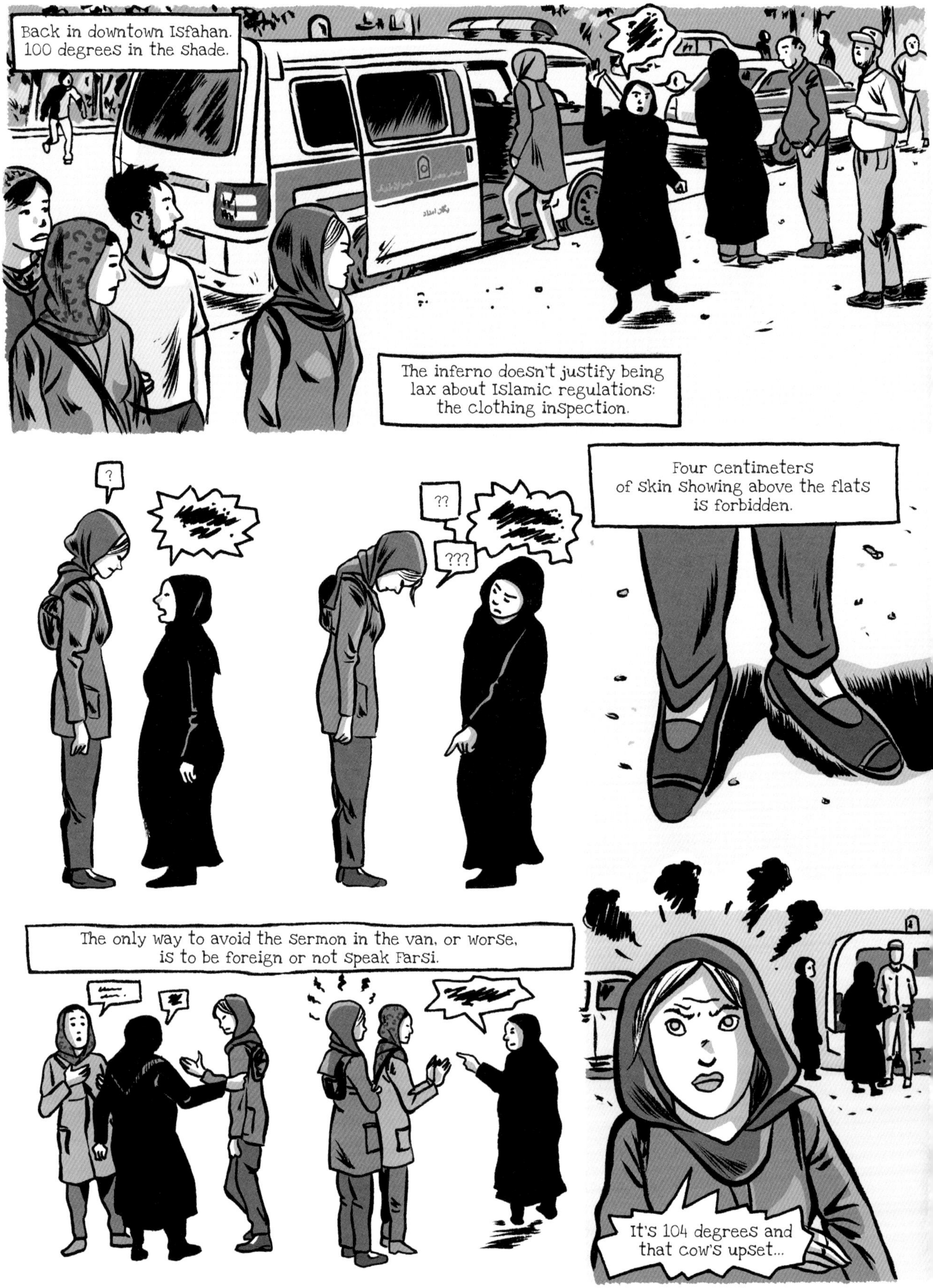

Back in downtown Isfahan. 100 degrees in the shade.
The inferno doesn't justify being lax about Islamic regulations: the clothing inspection.
?
??
???
Four centimeters of skin showing above the flats is forbidden.
The only way to avoid the sermon in the van, or worse, is to be foreign or not speak Farsi.
It's 104 degrees and that cow's upset...

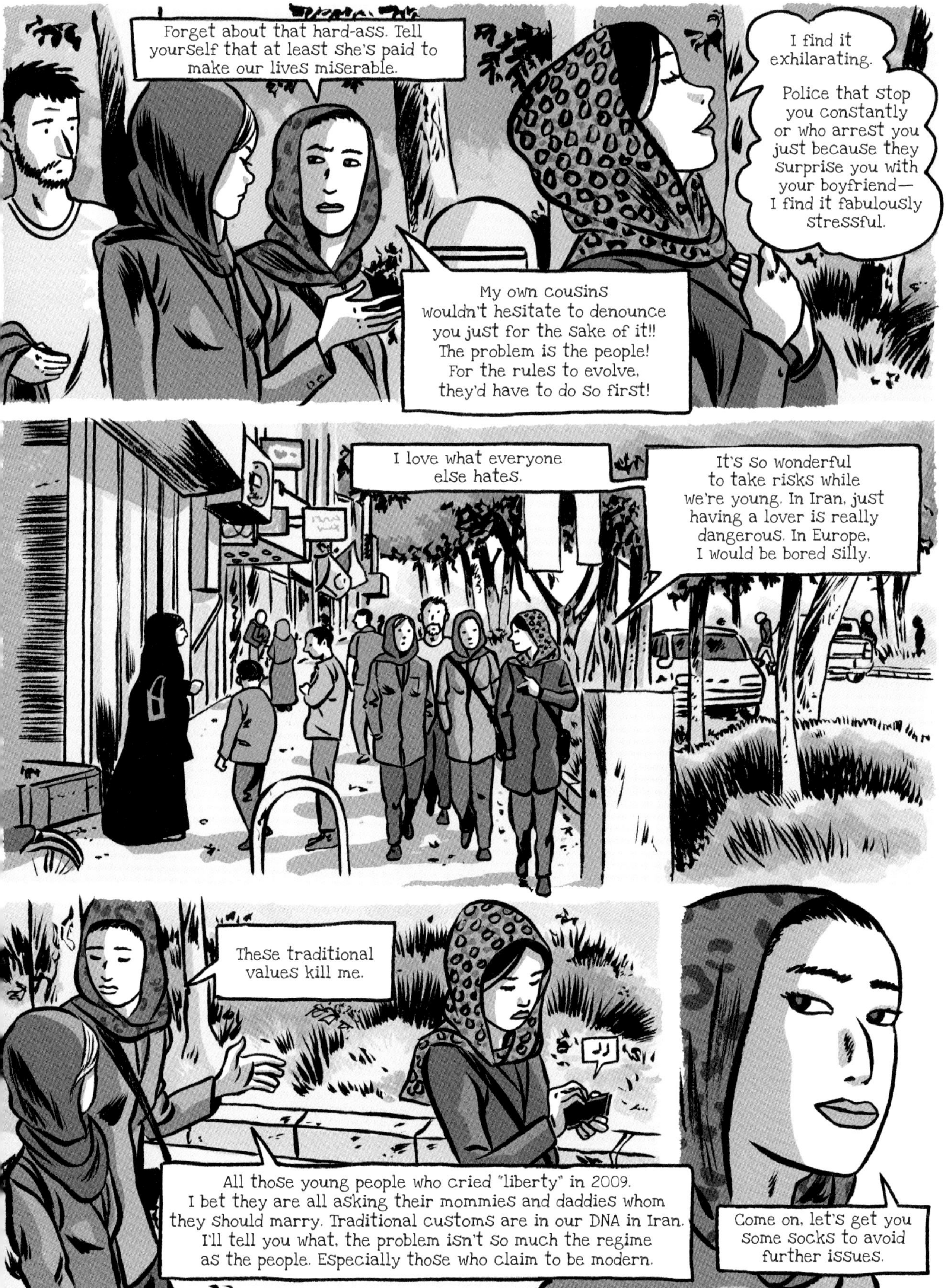
Forget about that hard-ass. Tell yourself that at least she's paid to make our lives miserable.
I find it exhilarating.
Police that stop you constantly or who arrest you just because they surprise you with your boyfriend— I find it fabulously stressful.
My own cousins wouldn't hesitate to denounce you just for the sake of it!! The problem is the people! For the rules to evolve, they'd have to do so first!
I love what everyone else hates.
It's so wonderful to take risks while we're young. In Iran, just having a lover is really dangerous. In Europe, I would be bored silly.
These traditional values kill me.
All those young people who cried "liberty" in 2009. I bet they are all asking their mommies and daddies whom they should marry. Traditional customs are in our DNA in Iran. I'll tell you what, the problem isn't so much the regime as the people. Especially those who claim to be modern.
Come on, let's get you some socks to avoid further issues.

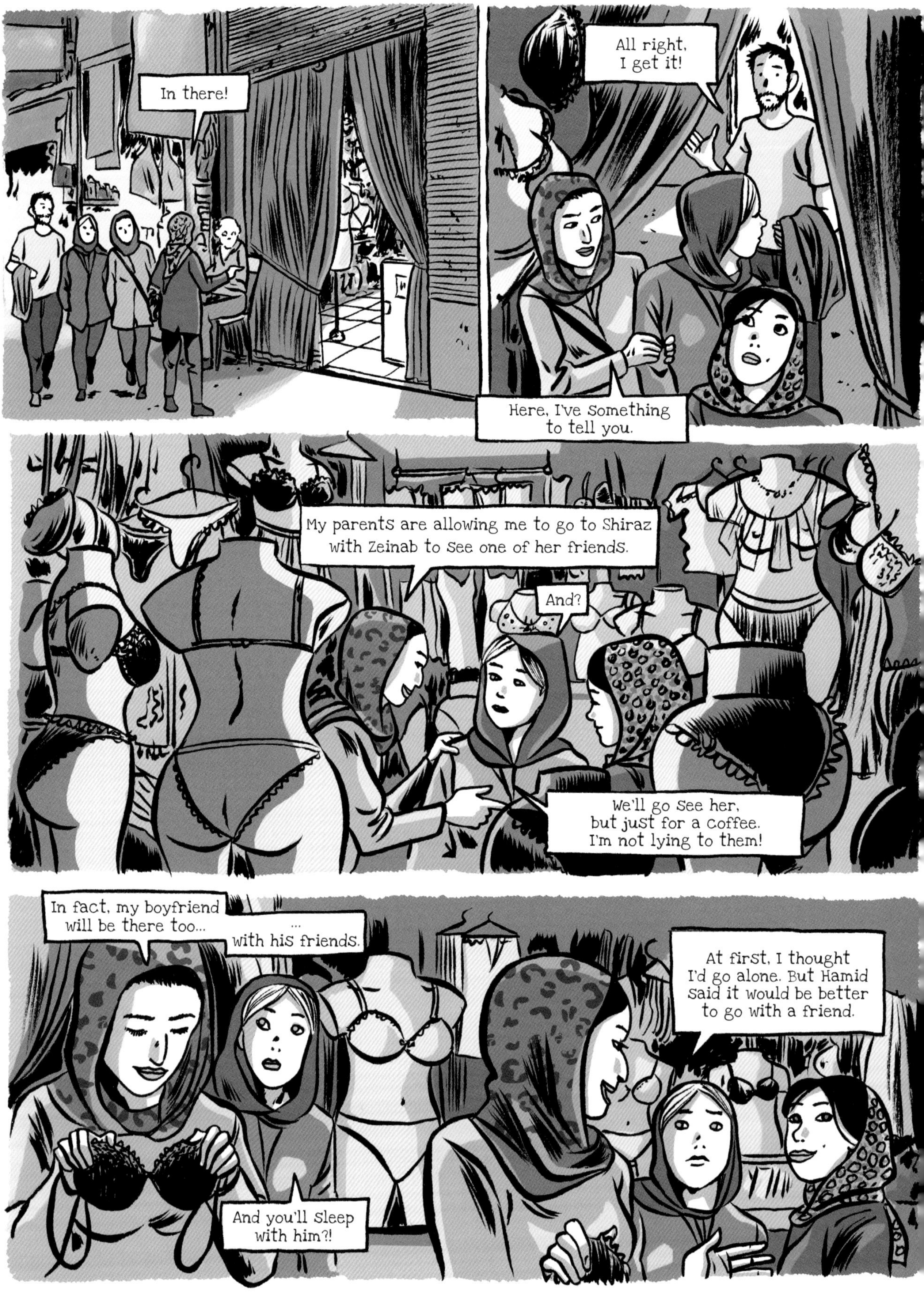

In there!
All right, I get it!
Here, I've something to tell you.
My parents are allowing me to go to Shiraz with Zeinab to see one of her friends.
And?
We'll go see her, but just for a coffee. I'm not lying to them!
In fact, my boyfriend will be there too...
... with his friends.
And you'll sleep with him?!
At first, I thought I'd go alone. But Hamid said it would be better to go with a friend.

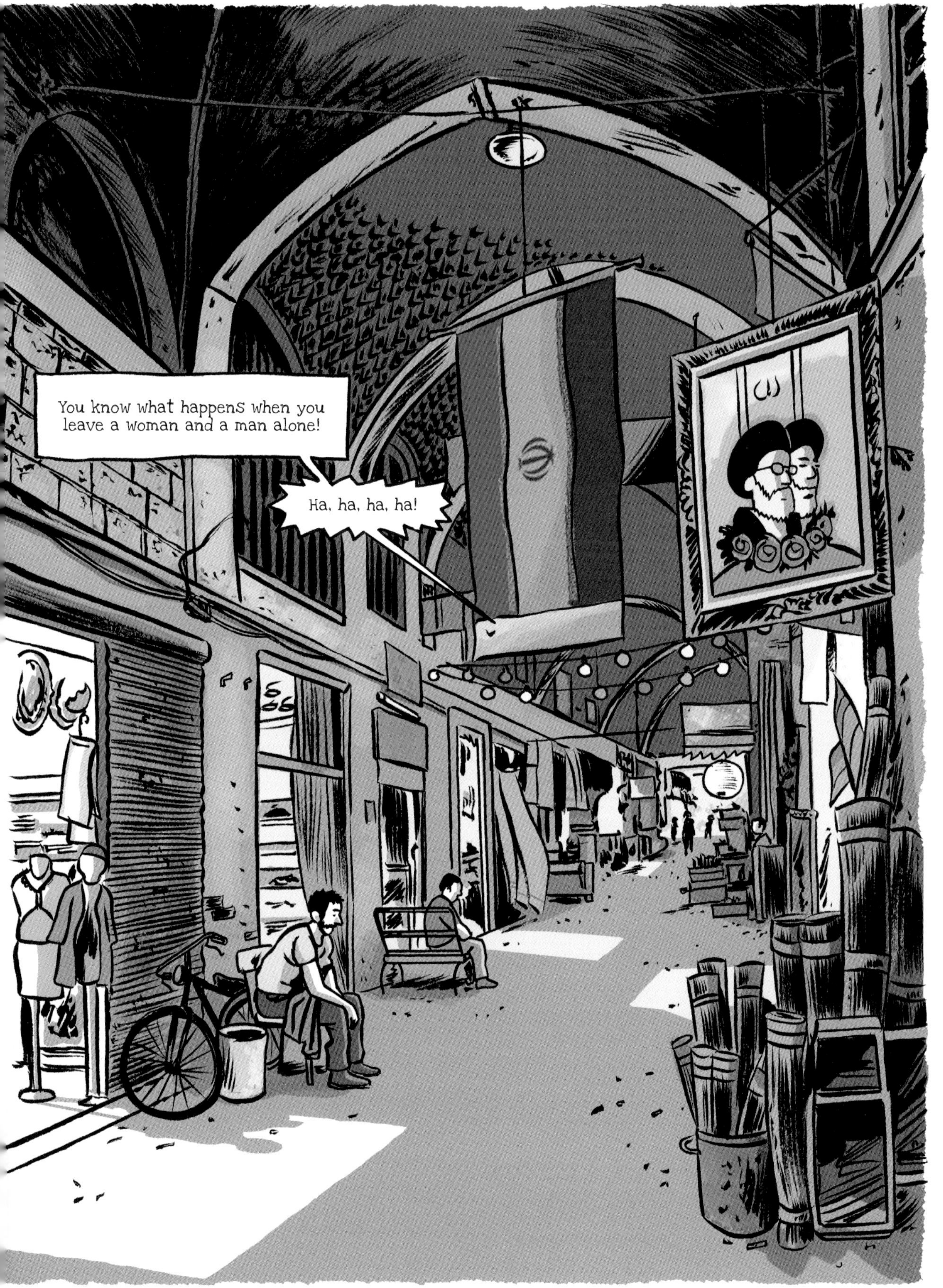

You know what happens when you leave a woman and a man alone!
Ha, ha, ha, ha!

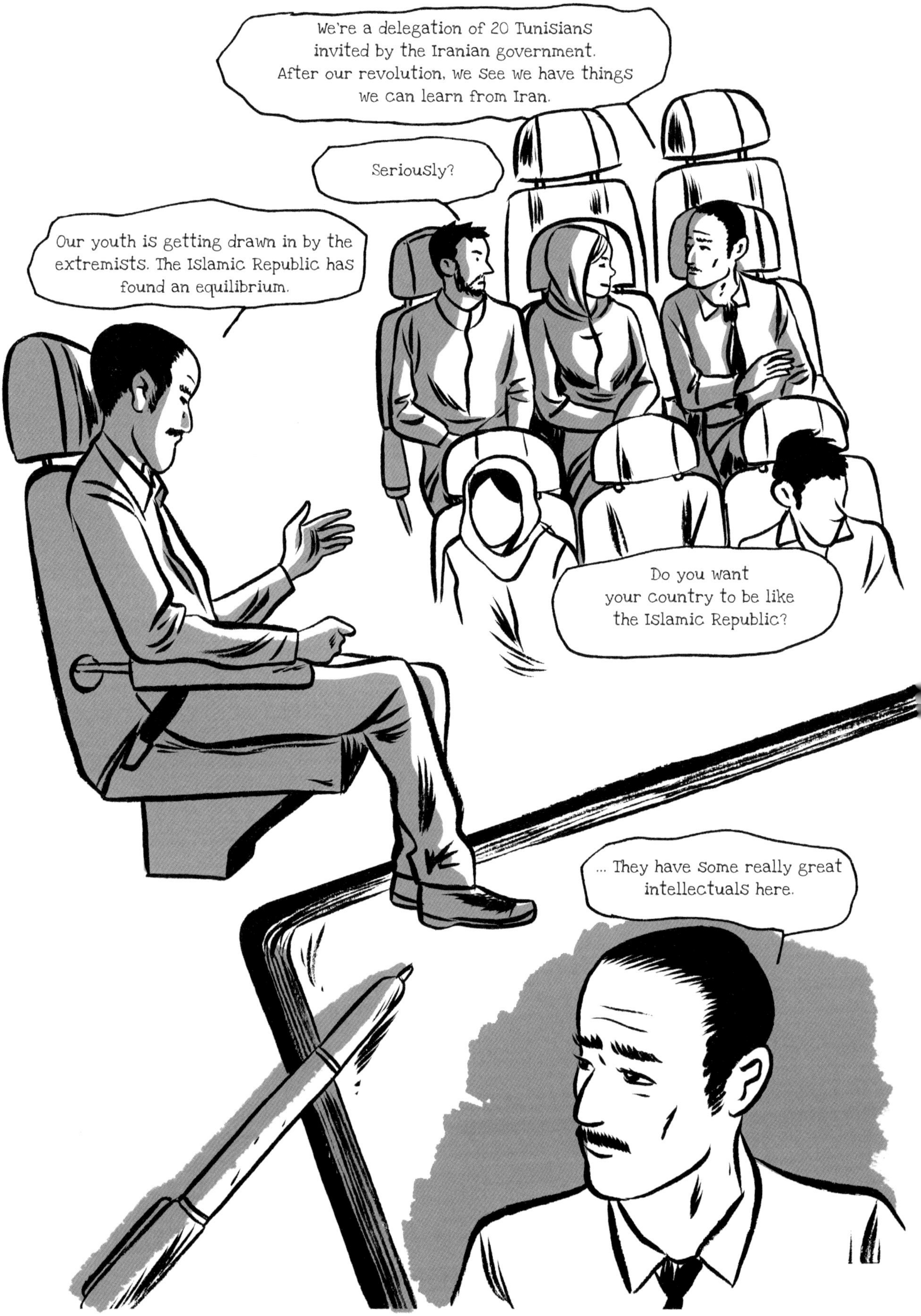
We're a delegation of 20 Tunisians invited by the Iranian government. After our revolution, we see we have things we can learn from Iran.
Seriously?
Our youth is getting drawn in by the extremists. The Islamic Republic has found an equilibrium.
Do you want your country to be like the Islamic Republic?
... They have some really great intellectuals here.

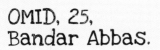

OMID, 25,
Bandar Abbas.

Omid invited us to his
place. He spoke to us
in perfect English.

His mother did
not hear our
conversation.

Luckily.

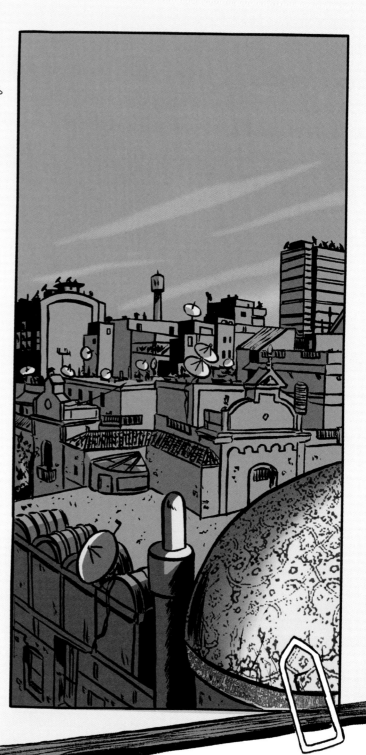

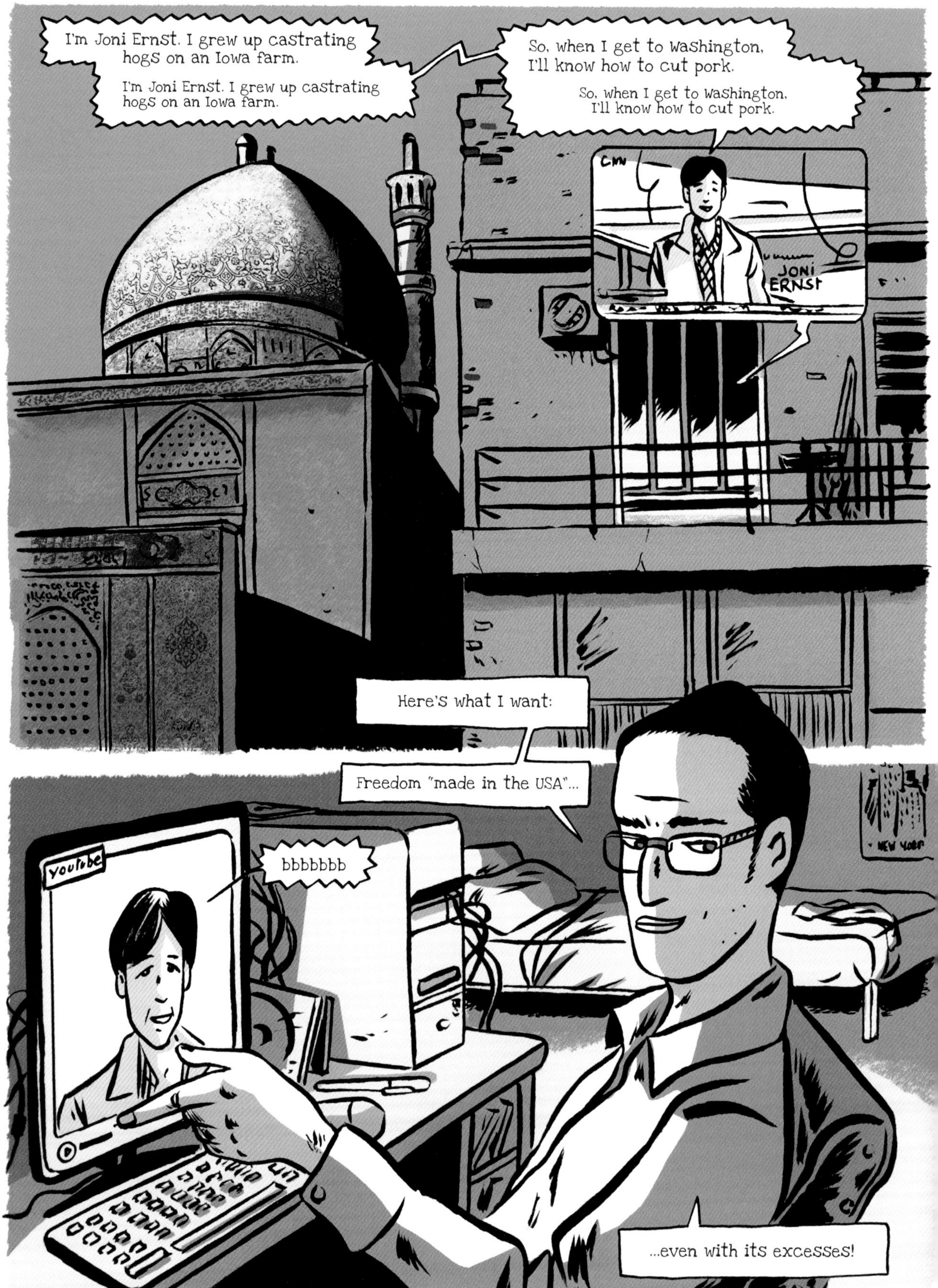
I'm Joni Ernst. I grew up castrating hogs on an Iowa farm.
I'm Joni Ernst. I grew up castrating hogs on an Iowa farm.
So, when I get to Washington, I'll know how to cut pork.
So, when I get to Washington, I'll know how to cut pork.
JONI ERNST
Here's what I want:
Freedom "made in the USA"...
youtube
bbbbbbb
...even with its excesses!

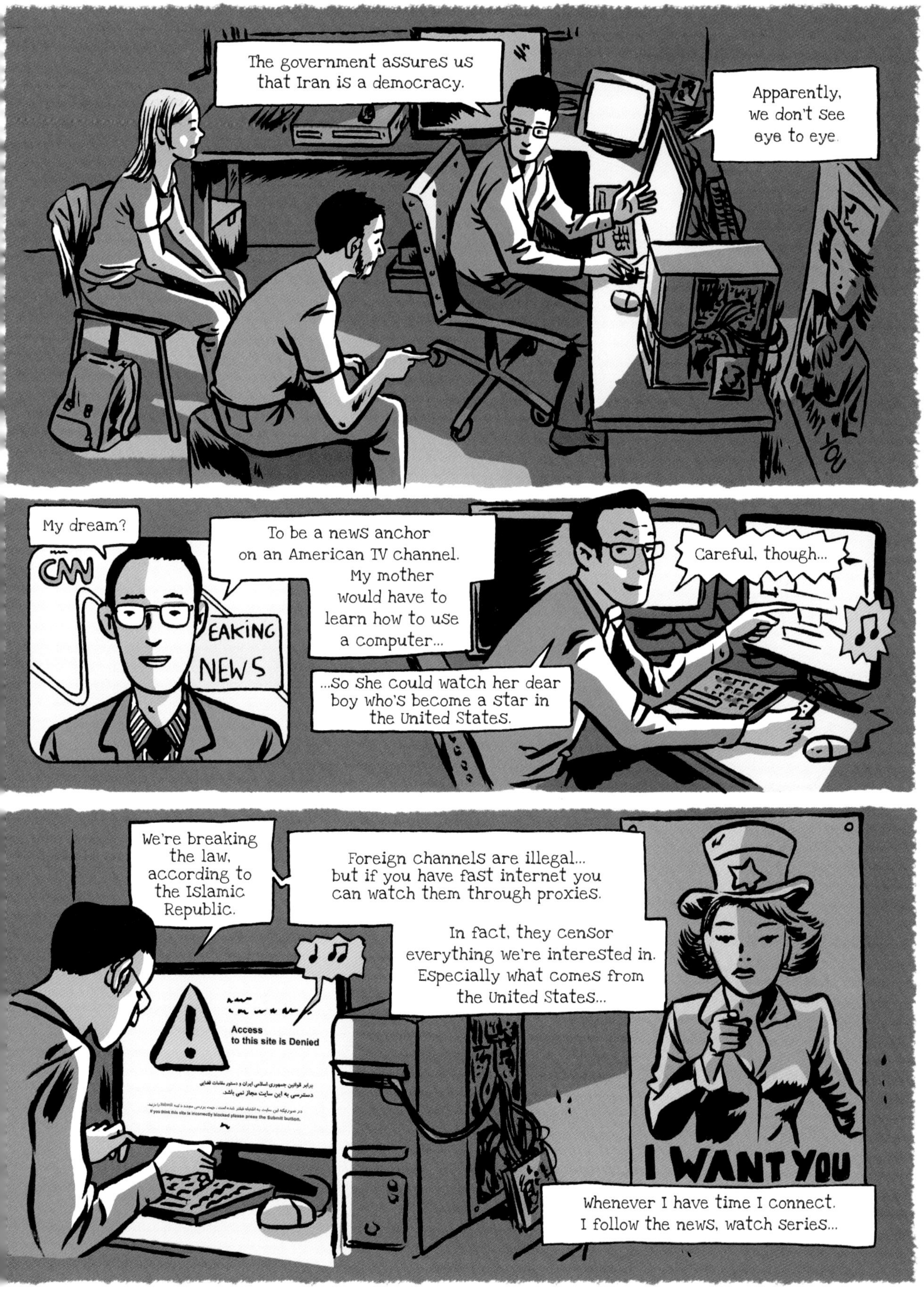
The government assures us that Iran is a democracy.
Apparently, we don't see eye to eye.
I WANT YOU
My dream?
CNN
EAKING NEWS
To be a news anchor on an American TV channel. My mother would have to learn how to use a computer...
...So she could watch her dear boy who's become a star in the United States.
Careful, though...
We're breaking the law, according to the Islamic Republic.
Foreign channels are illegal... but if you have fast internet you can watch them through proxies.
In fact, they censor everything we're interested in. Especially what comes from the United States...
Access
to this site is Denied
برابر قوانین جمهوری اسلامی ایران و دستور مقامات قضایی
دسترسی به این سایت مجاز نمی باشد.
If you think this site is incorrectly blocked please press the Submit button.
I WANT YOU
Whenever I have time I connect. I follow the news, watch series...

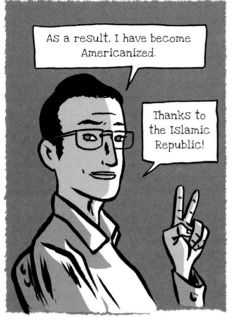

As a result, I have become Americanized.

Thanks to the Islamic Republic!

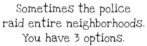

Sometimes the police raid entire neighborhoods. You have 3 options.

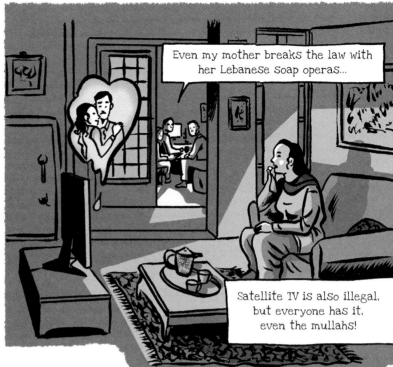

Even my mother breaks the law with her Lebanese soap operas...

Satellite TV is also illegal, but everyone has it, even the mullahs!

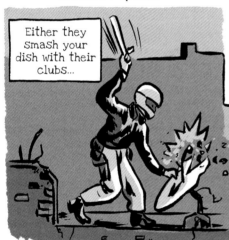

Either they smash your dish with their clubs...

or they throw it off the building.

Or they steal it.

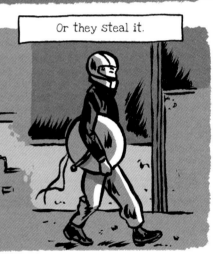

The next day, everyone buys a new one. I'm guessing it's a way to boost the economy.

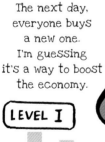

LEVEL I

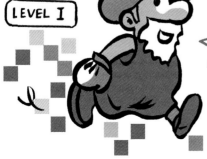

SUPER MOLIAH

WIN

30 Pts

Dishes have been illegal since 1994, but—and it was the head of state TV who confirmed this— almost 70% of the households own one.

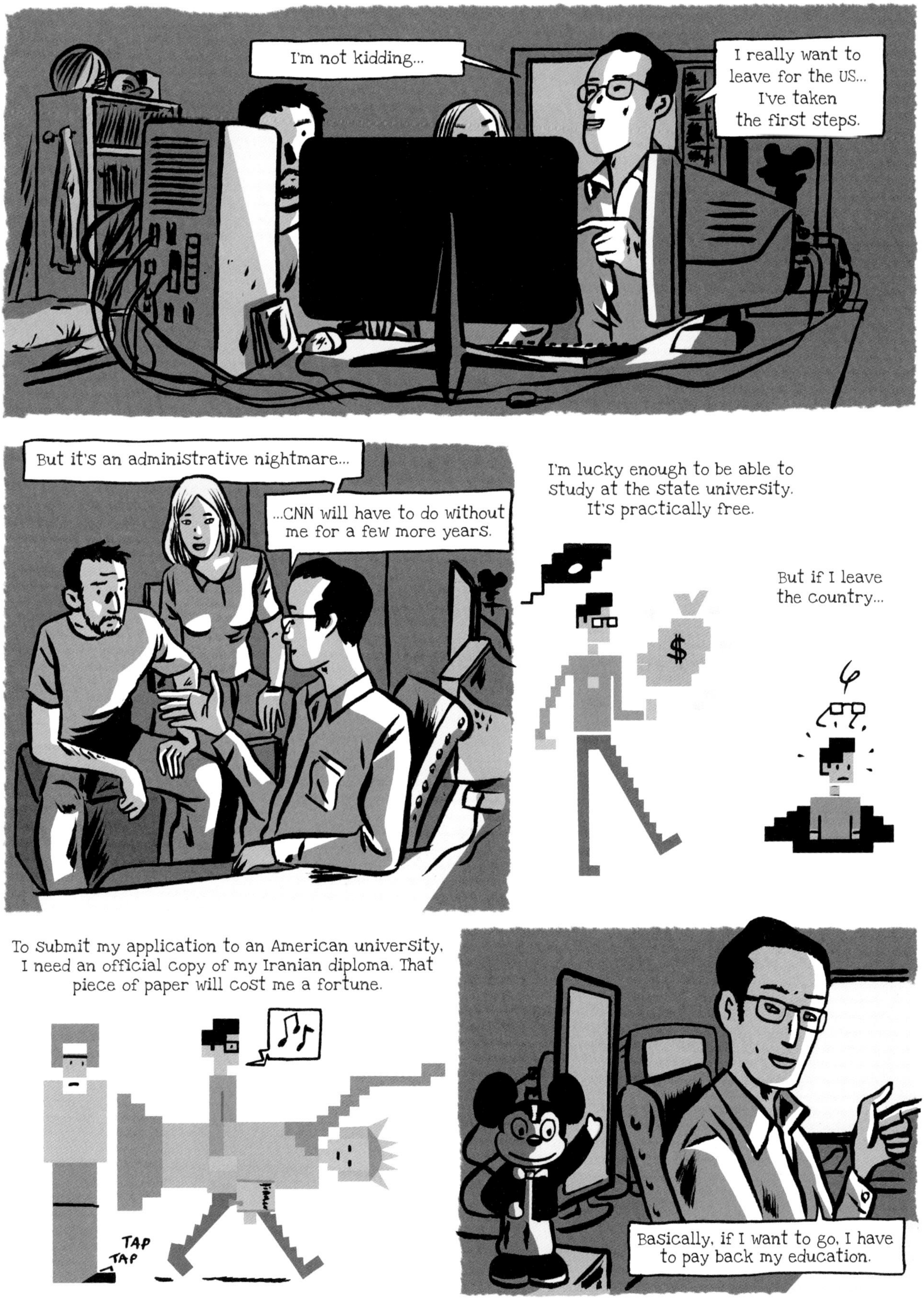
I'm not kidding...
I really want to leave for the US... I've taken the first steps.
But it's an administrative nightmare...
...CNN will have to do without me for a few more years.
I'm lucky enough to be able to study at the state university. It's practically free.
$
But if I leave the country...
To submit my application to an American university, I need an official copy of my Iranian diploma. That piece of paper will cost me a fortune.
TAP TAP
Basically, if I want to go, I have to pay back my education.

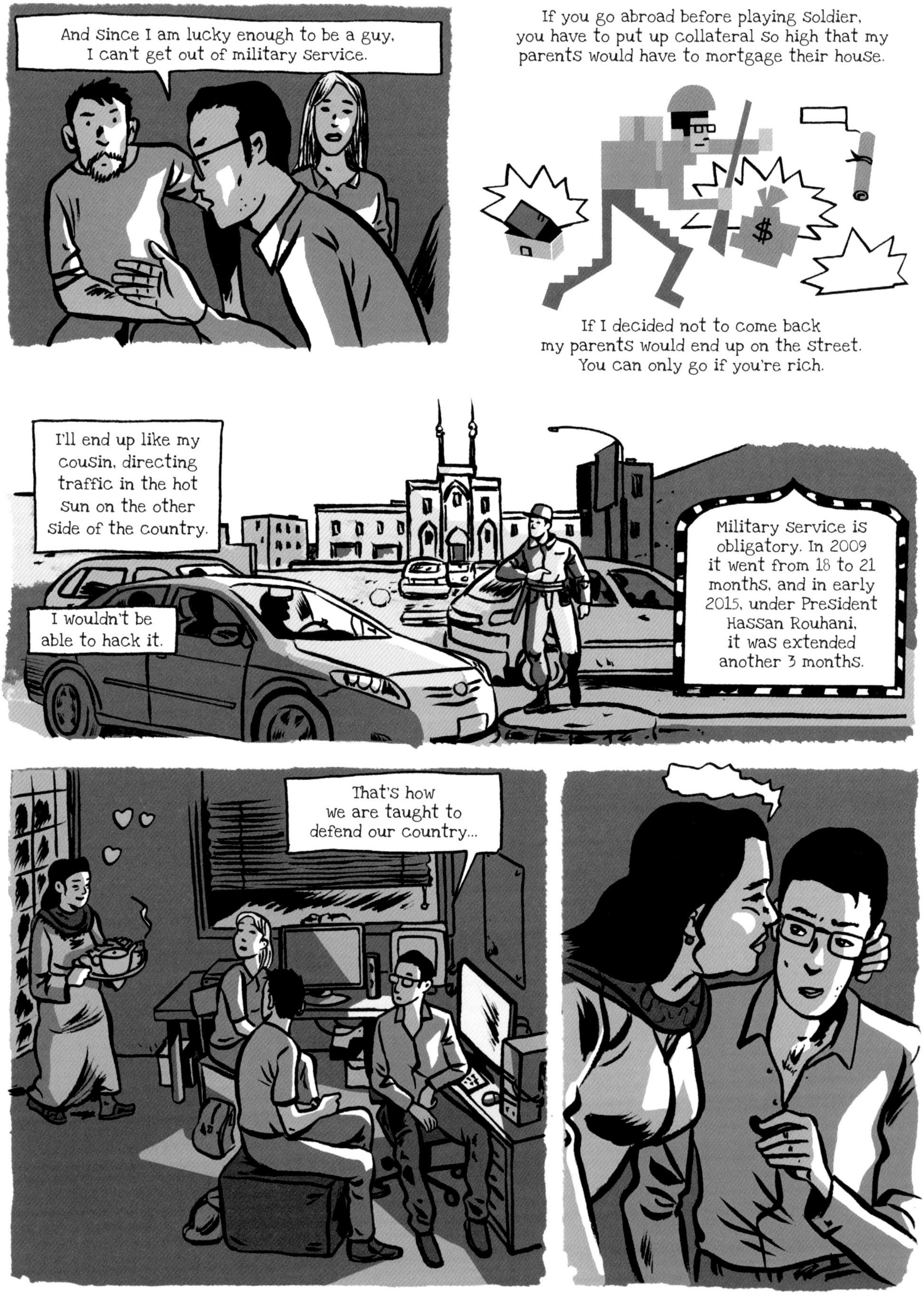
And since I am lucky enough to be a guy, I can't get out of military service.
If you go abroad before playing soldier, you have to put up collateral so high that my parents would have to mortgage their house.
$
If I decided not to come back my parents would end up on the street. You can only go if you're rich.
I'll end up like my cousin, directing traffic in the hot sun on the other side of the country.
I wouldn't be able to hack it.
Military service is obligatory. In 2009 it went from 18 to 21 months, and in early 2015, under President Hassan Rouhani, it was extended another 3 months.
That's how we are taught to defend our country...

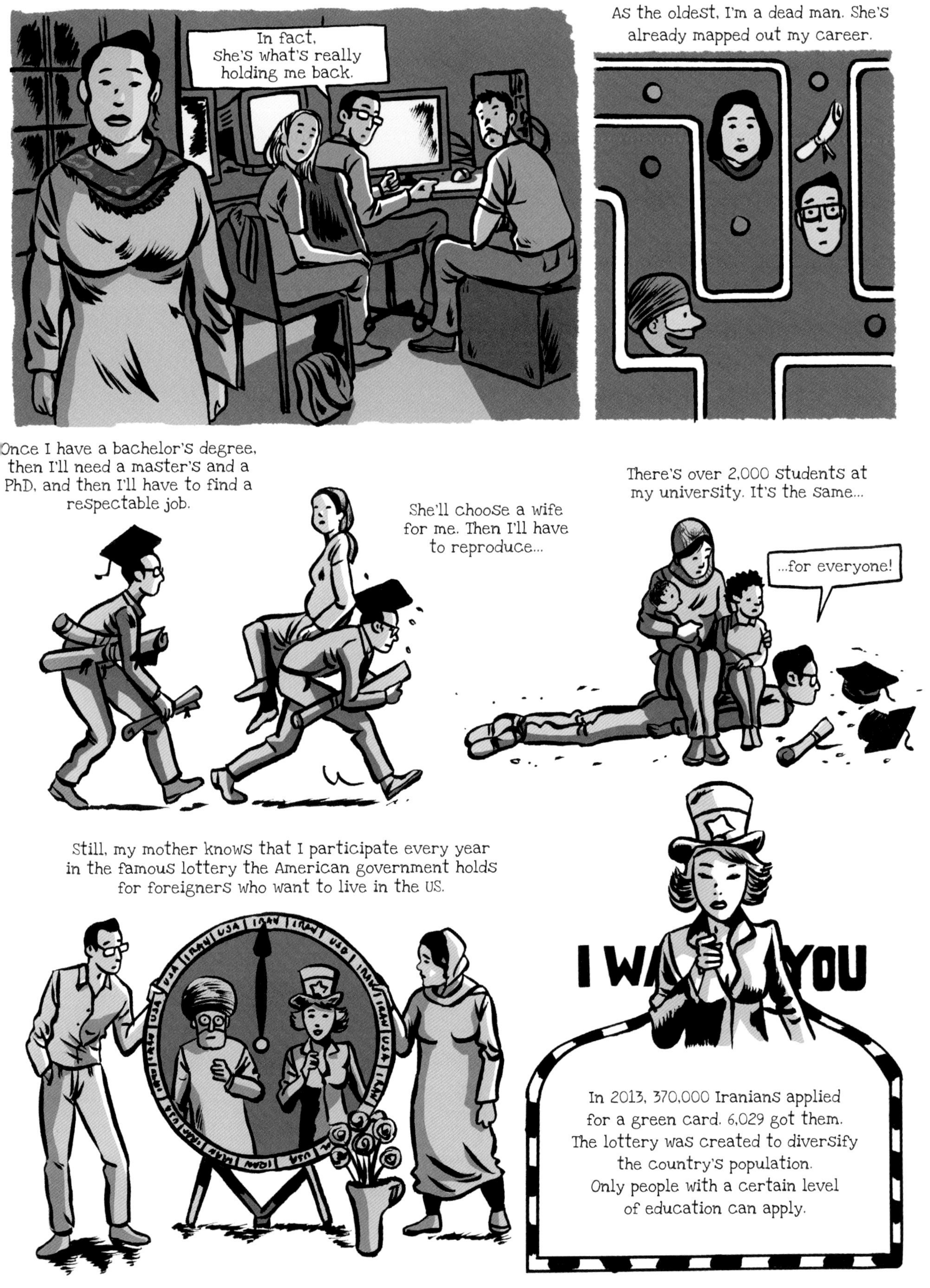
In fact, she's what's really holding me back.
As the oldest, I'm a dead man. She's already mapped out my career.
Once I have a bachelor's degree, then I'll need a master's and a PhD, and then I'll have to find a respectable job.
She'll choose a wife for me. Then I'll have to reproduce...
There's over 2,000 students at my university. It's the same...
...for everyone!
Still, my mother knows that I participate every year in the famous lottery the American government holds for foreigners who want to live in the US.
In 2013, 370,000 Iranians applied for a green card. 6,029 got them. The lottery was created to diversify the country's population. Only people with a certain level of education can apply.

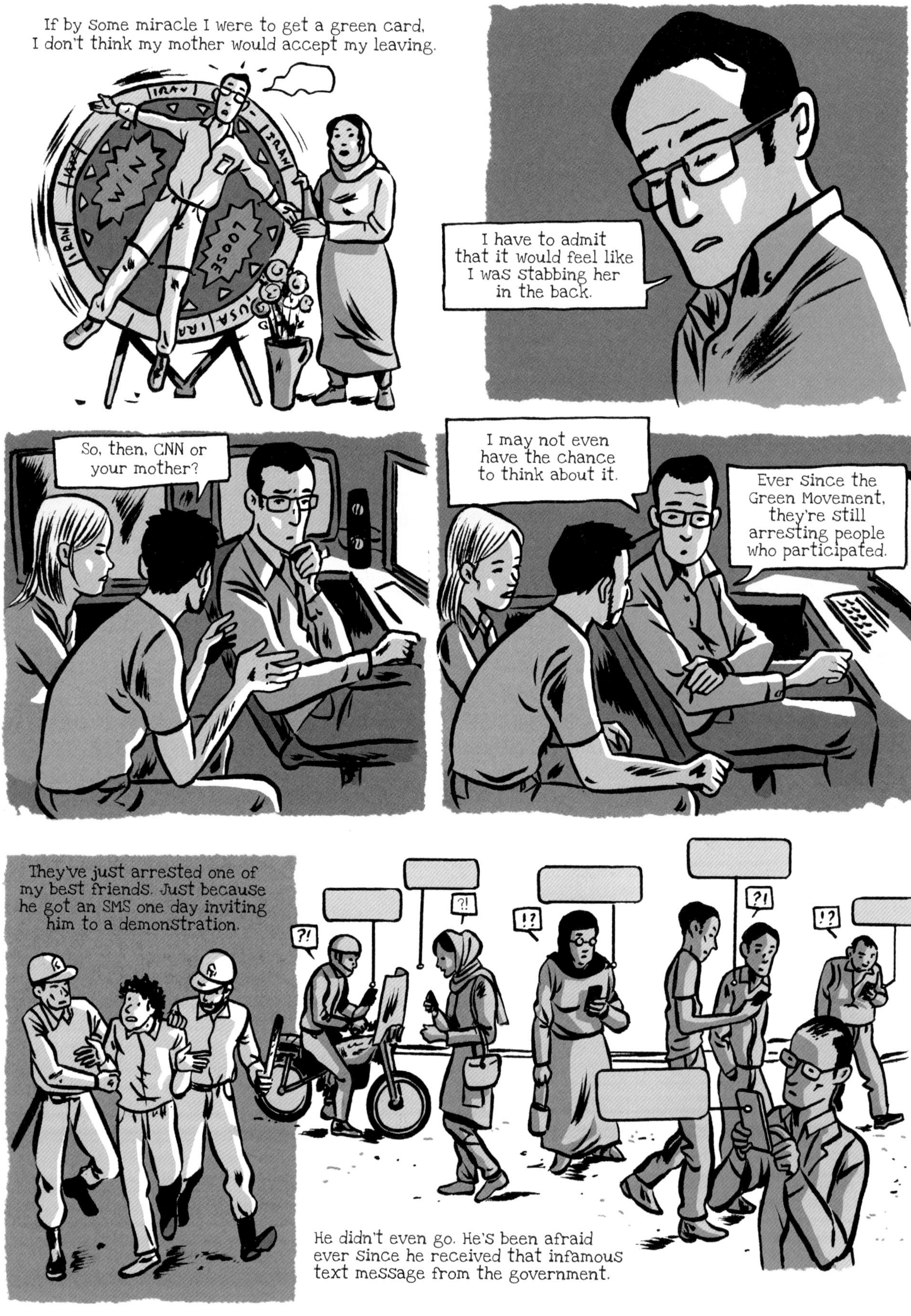
If by some miracle I were to get a green card, I don't think my mother would accept my leaving.
IRAN
IRAN
IRAN
USA
IRAN
WIN
LOOSE
I have to admit that it would feel like I was stabbing her in the back.
So, then, CNN or your mother?
I may not even have the chance to think about it.
Ever since the Green Movement, they're still arresting people who participated.
They've just arrested one of my best friends. Just because he got an SMS one day inviting him to a demonstration.
?!
?!
!?
?!
!?
He didn't even go. He's been afraid ever since he received that infamous text message from the government.

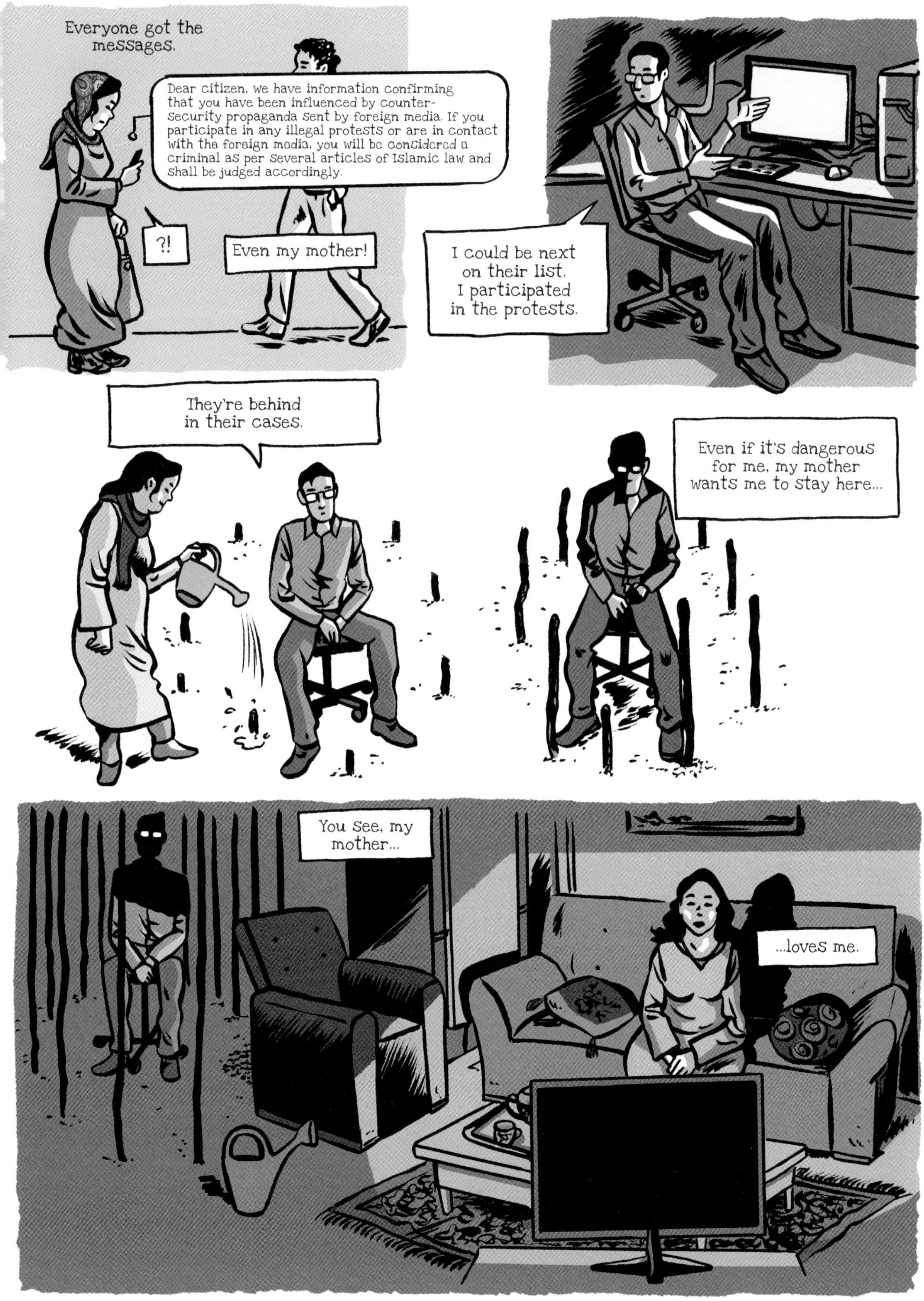
Everyone got the messages.
Dear citizen, we have information confirming that you have been influenced by counter-security propaganda sent by foreign media. If you participate in any illegal protests or are in contact with the foreign media, you will be considered a criminal as per several articles of Islamic law and shall be judged accordingly.
?!
Even my mother!
I could be next on their list. I participated in the protests.
They're behind in their cases.
Even if it's dangerous for me, my mother wants me to stay here...
You see, my mother...
...loves me.

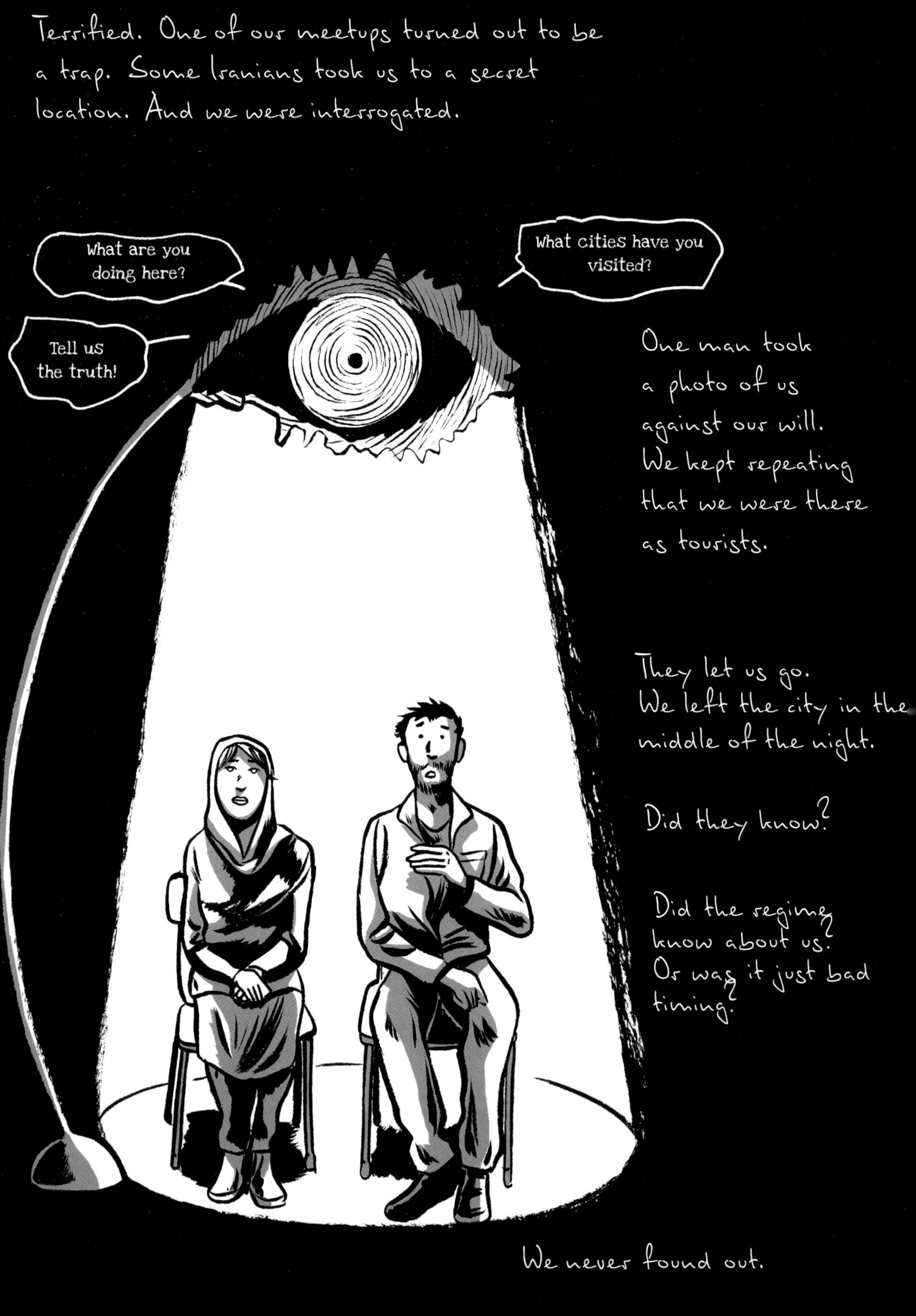
Terrified. One of our meetups turned out to be a trap. Some Iranians took us to a secret location. And we were interrogated.
What are you doing here?
What cities have you visited?
Tell us the truth!
One man took a photo of us against our will. We kept repeating that we were there as tourists.
They let us go. We left the city in the middle of the night.
Did they know?
Did the regime know about us? Or was it just bad timing?
We never found out.

ASHEM, 20 and NIMA, 20,
Yazd.

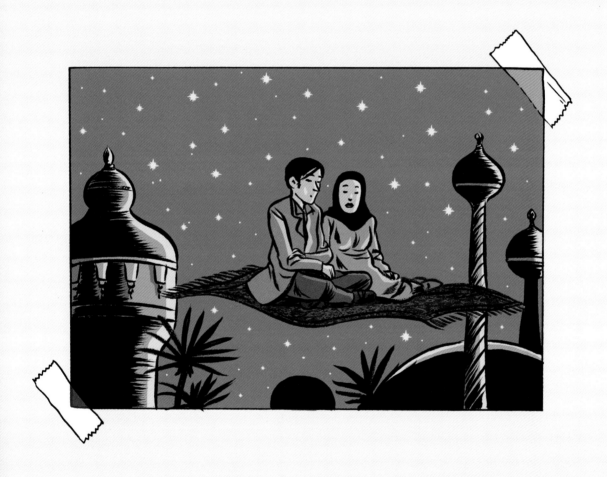

Like so many Iranians, they met at university.

And like so many Iranians,
they don't need the regime to ruin their lives.

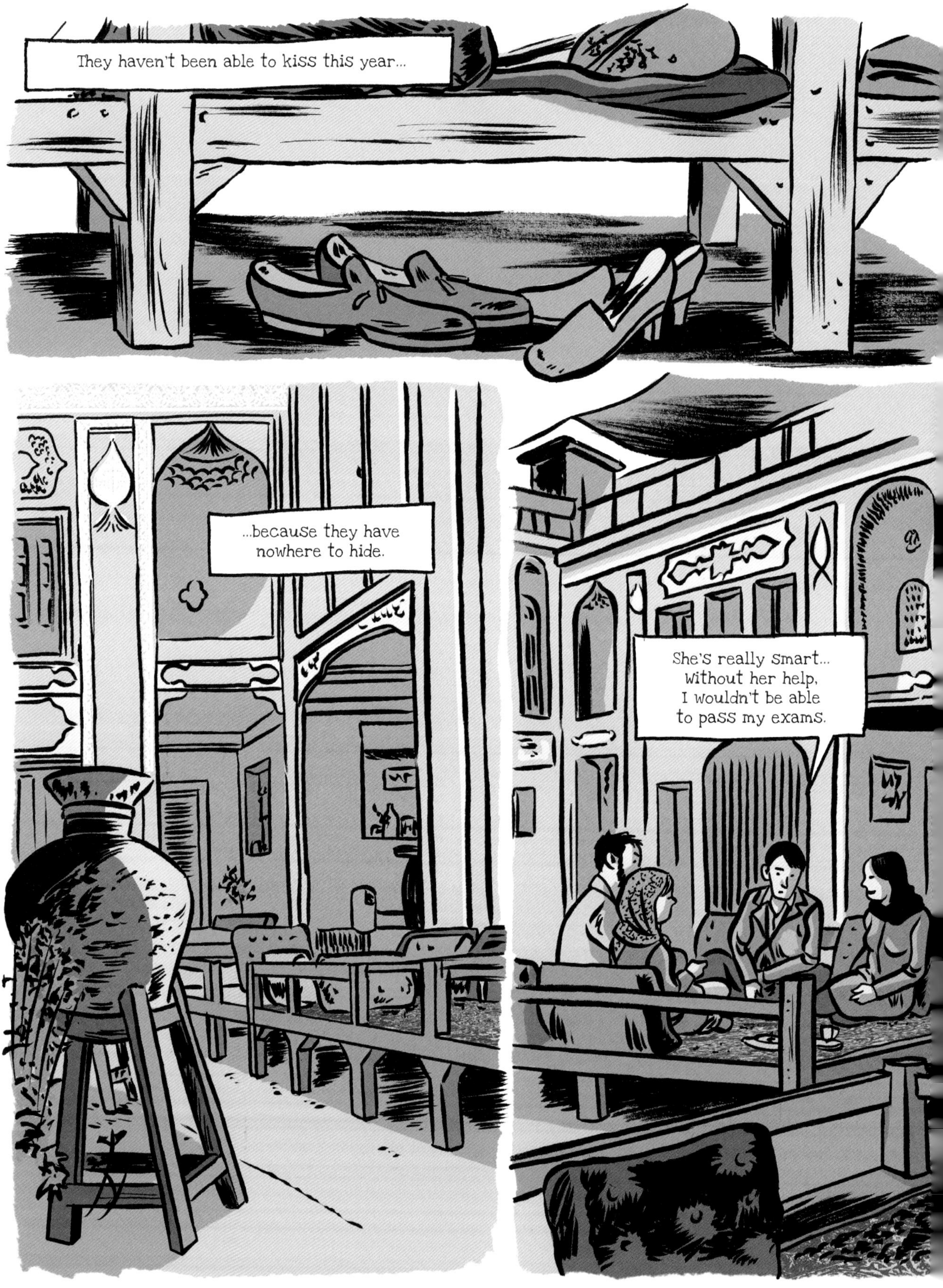
They haven't been able to kiss this year...
...because they have nowhere to hide.
She's really smart... Without her help, I wouldn't be able to pass my exams.

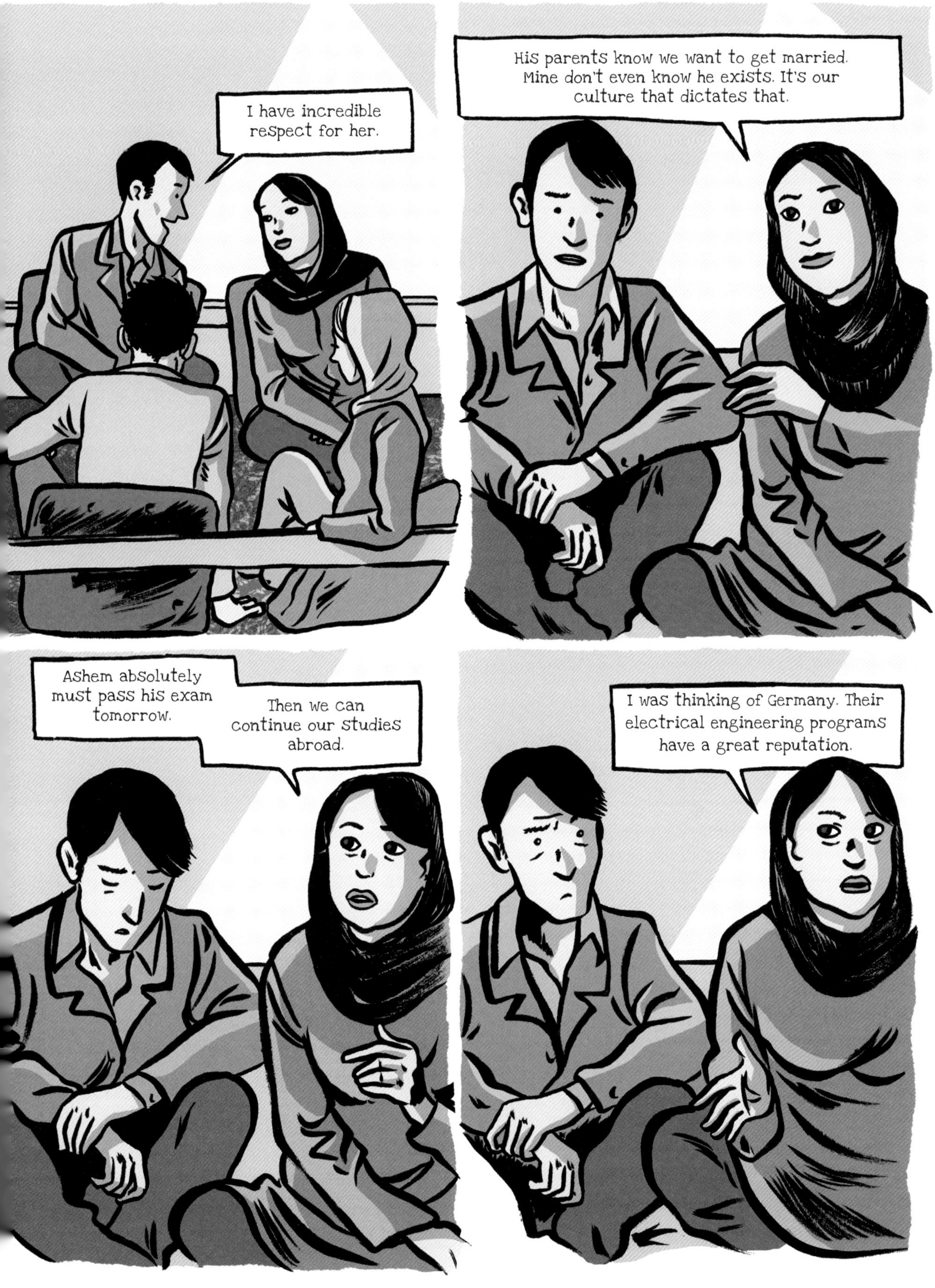
I have incredible respect for her.
His parents know we want to get married. Mine don't even know he exists. It's our culture that dictates that.
Ashem absolutely must pass his exam tomorrow.
Then we can continue our studies abroad.
I was thinking of Germany. Their electrical engineering programs have a great reputation.

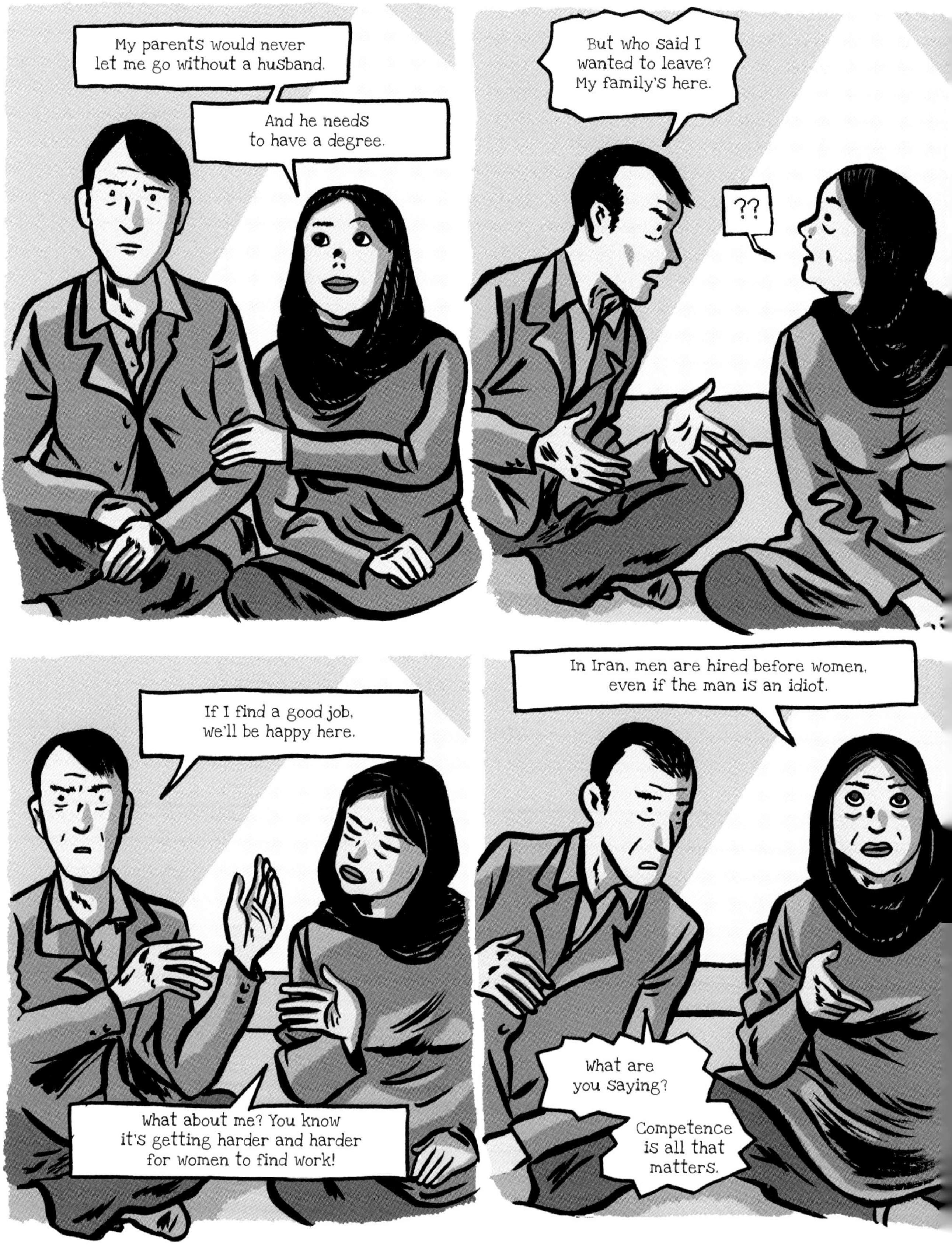
My parents would never let me go without a husband.
And he needs to have a degree.
But who said I wanted to leave? My family's here.
??
If I find a good job, we'll be happy here.
What about me? You know it's getting harder and harder for women to find work!
In Iran, men are hired before women, even if the man is an idiot.
What are you saying?
Competence is all that matters.

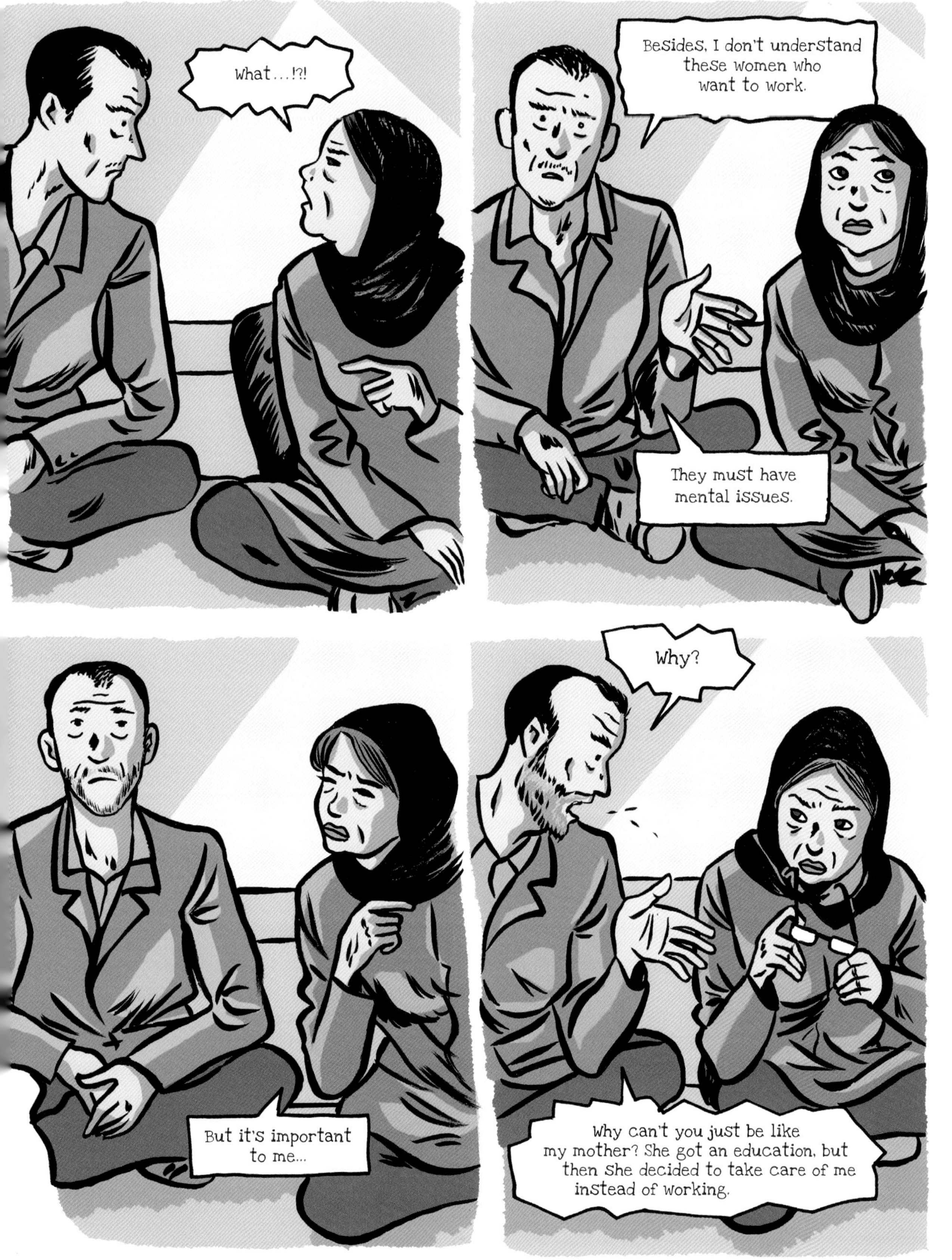

What...!?!
Besides, I don't understand these women who want to work.
They must have mental issues.
But it's important to me...
Why?
Why can't you just be like my mother? She got an education, but then she decided to take care of me instead of working.

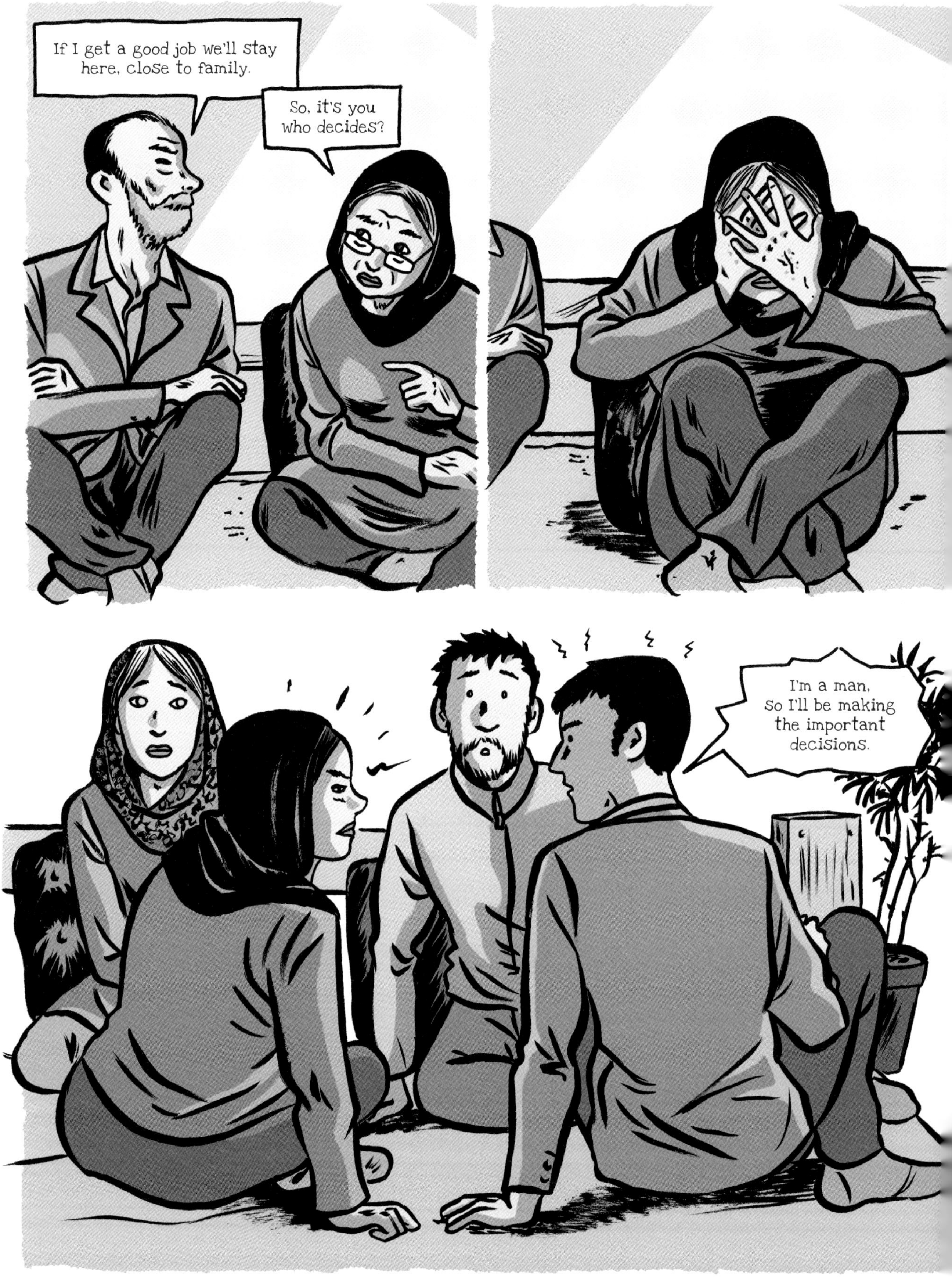
If I get a good job we'll stay here, close to family.
So, it's you who decides?
I'm a man, so I'll be making the important decisions.

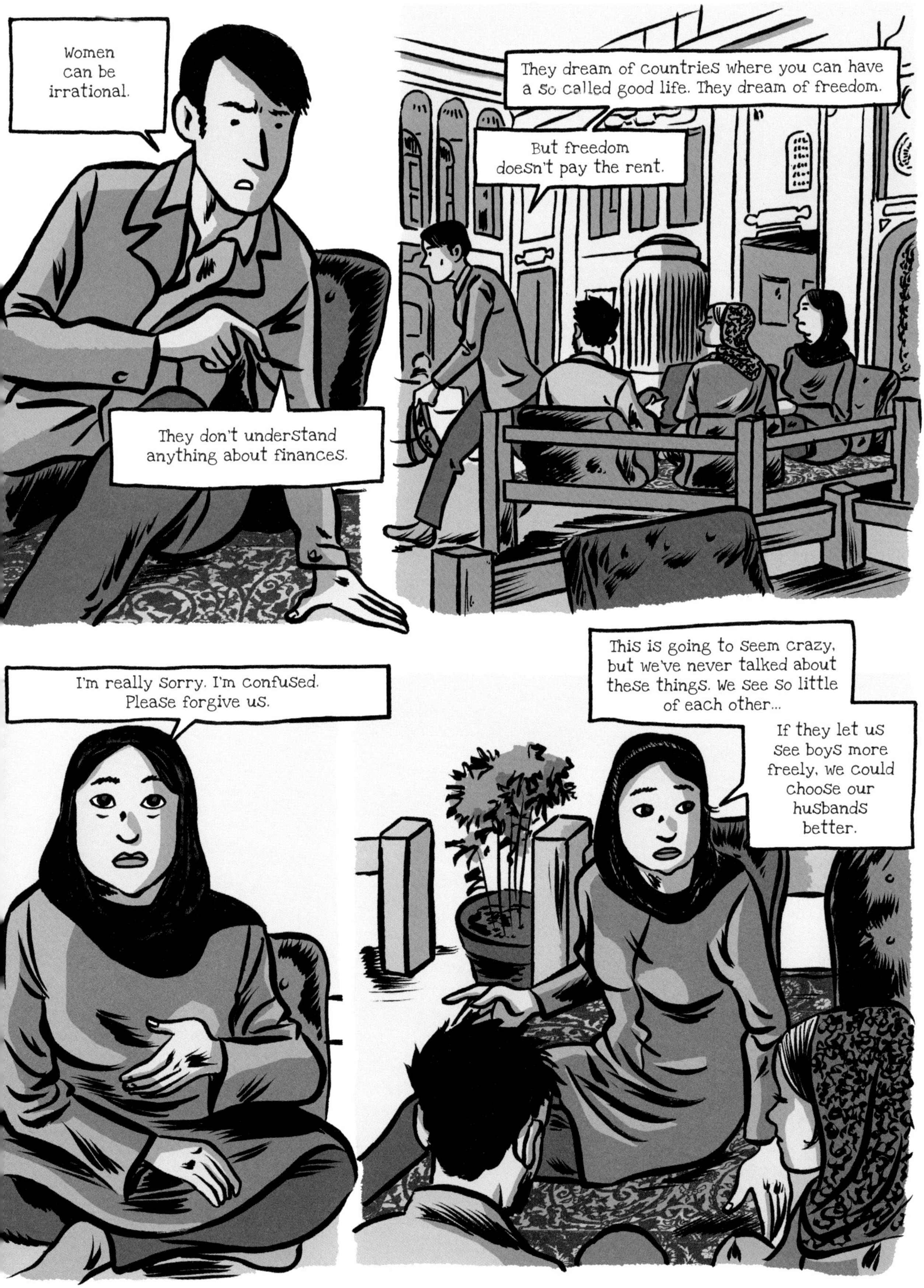
Women can be irrational.
They don't understand anything about finances.
They dream of countries where you can have a so called good life. They dream of freedom.
But freedom doesn't pay the rent.
I'm really sorry. I'm confused. Please forgive us.
This is going to seem crazy, but we've never talked about these things. We see so little of each other...
If they let us see boys more freely, we could choose our husbands better.

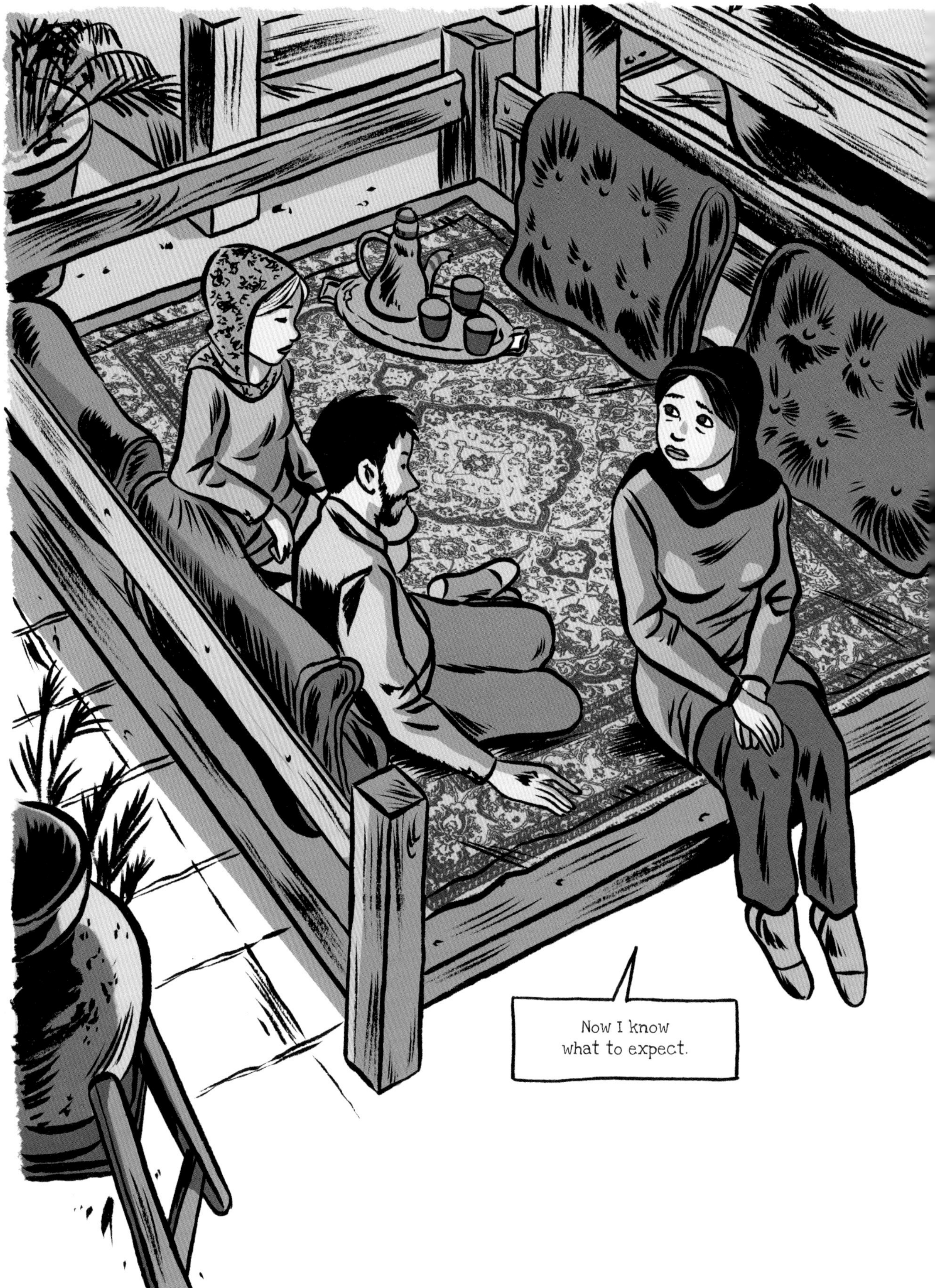
Now I know
what to expect.

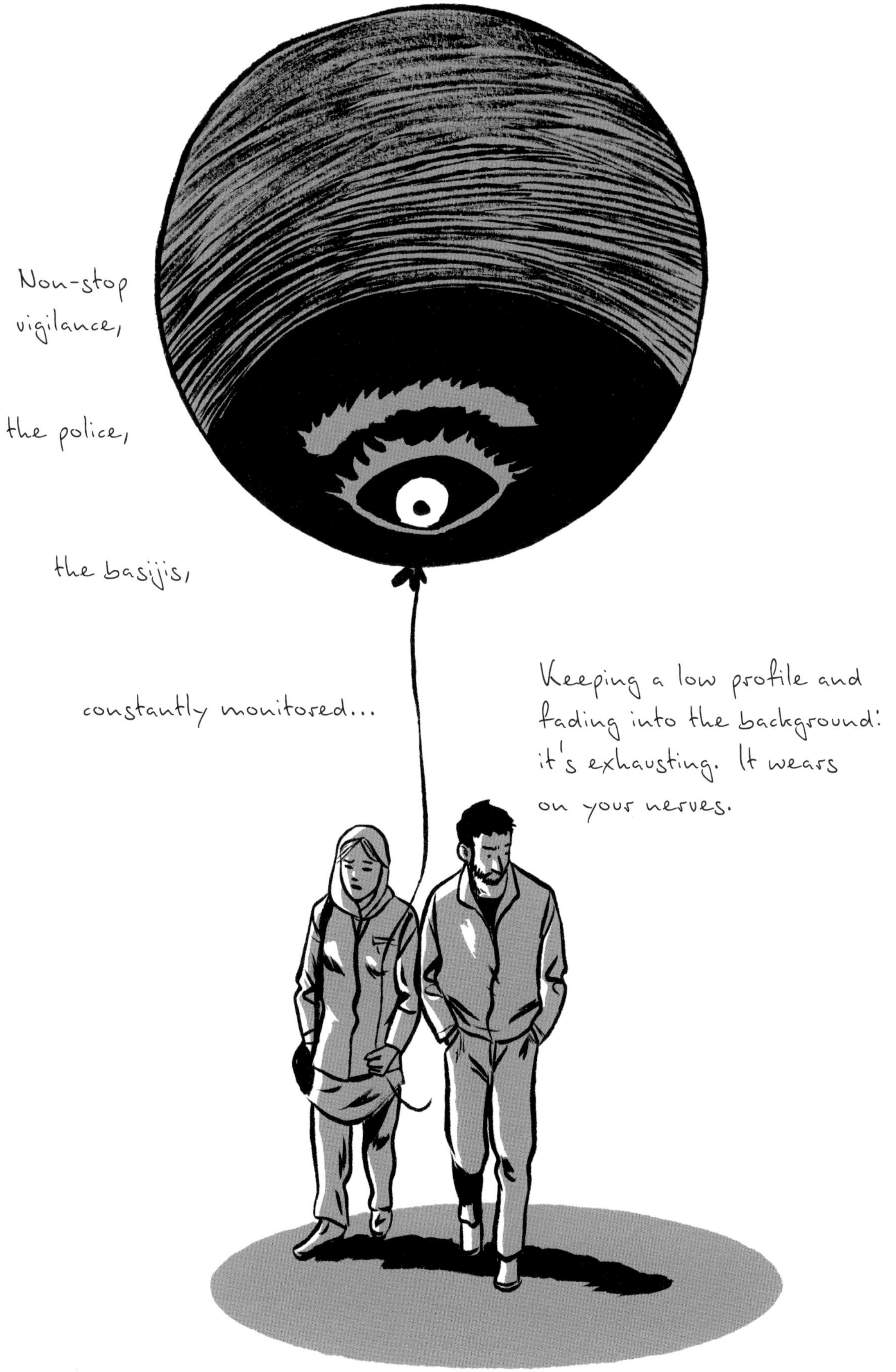
Non-stop vigilance,
the police,
the basijis,
constantly monitored...
Keeping a low profile and fading into the background: it's exhausting. It wears on your nerves.

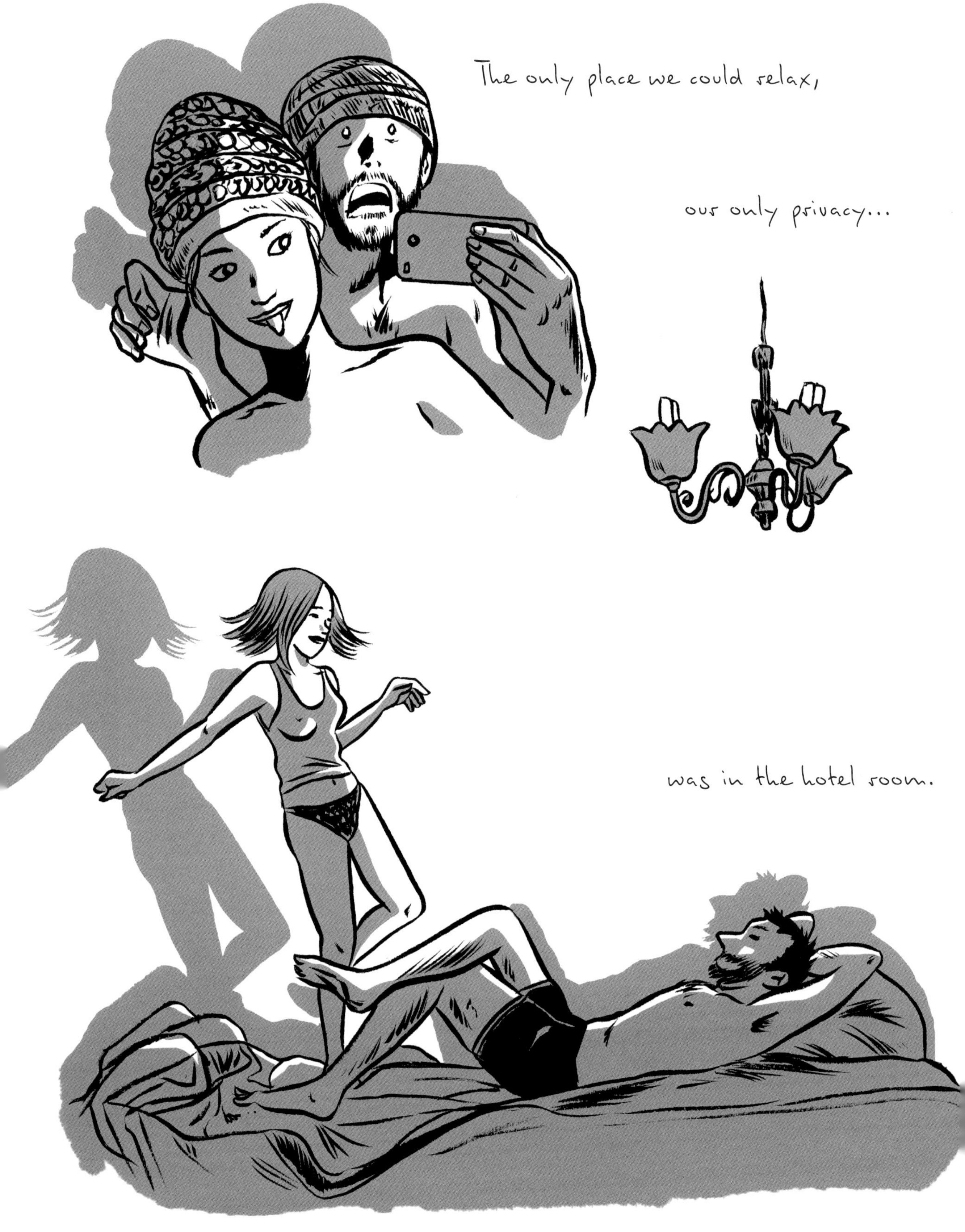
The only place we could relax,
our only privacy...
was in the hotel room.

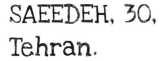

SAEEDEH, 30,
Tehran.

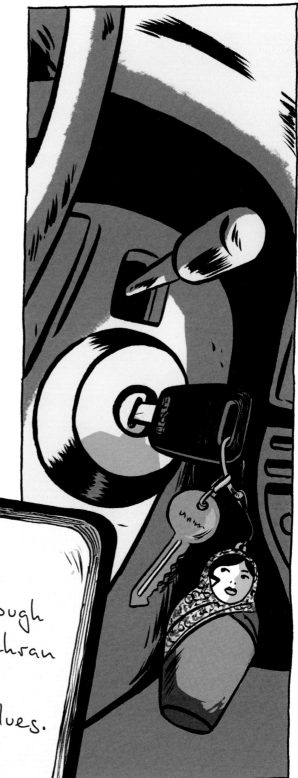

She was naïve enough
to think that in Tehran
she could get away
from traditional values.

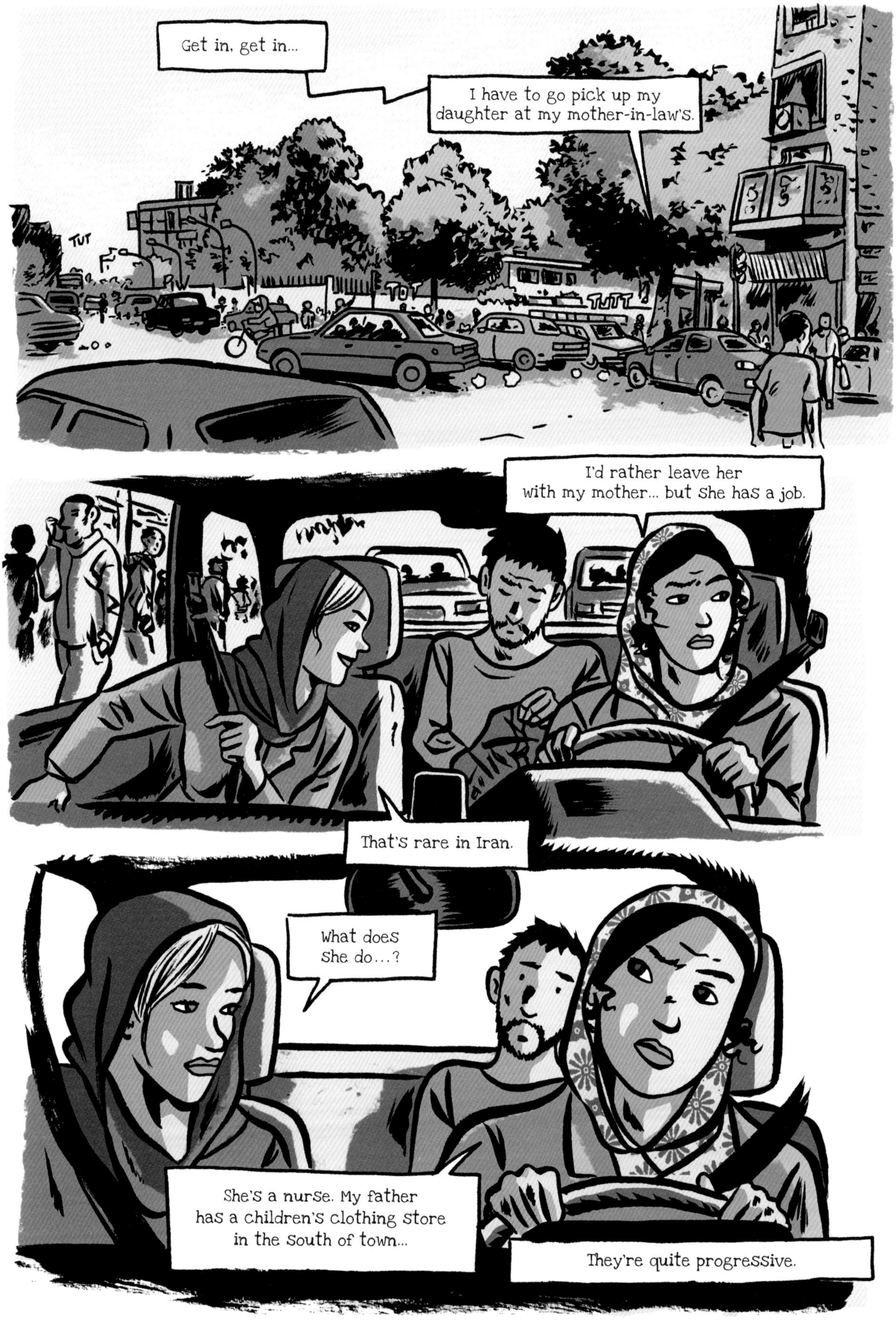
Get in, get in...
I have to go pick up my daughter at my mother-in-law's.
TUT
TUT
TUTT
I'd rather leave her with my mother... but she has a job.
That's rare in Iran.
What does she do...?
She's a nurse. My father has a children's clothing store in the south of town...
They're quite progressive.

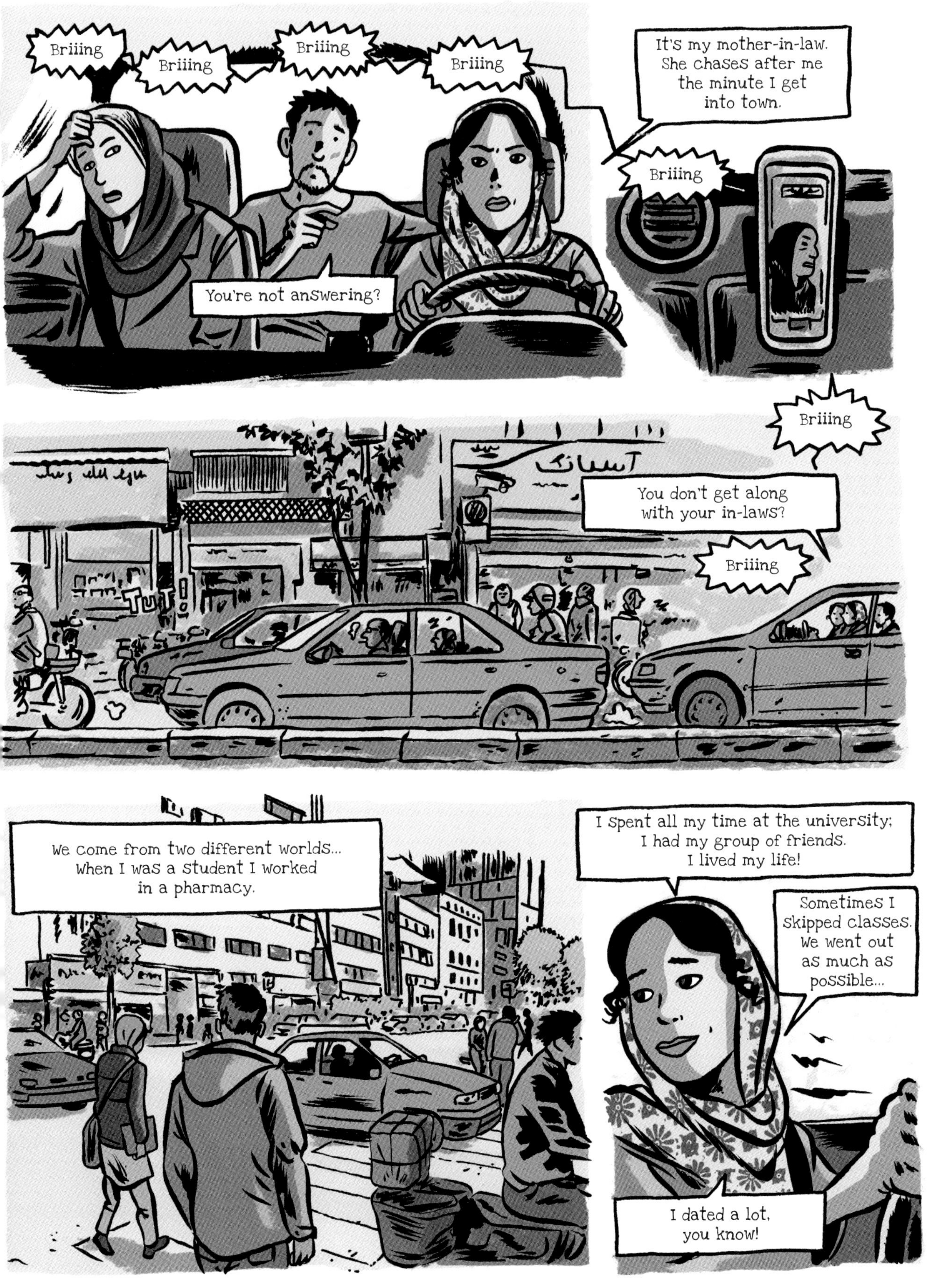
Briiing
Briiing
Briiing
Briiing
You're not answering?
It's my mother-in-law. She chases after me the minute I get into town.
Briiing
Briiing
You don't get along with your in-laws?
Briiing
We come from two different worlds... When I was a student I worked in a pharmacy.
I spent all my time at the university; I had my group of friends. I lived my life!
Sometimes I skipped classes. We went out as much as possible...
I dated a lot, you know!

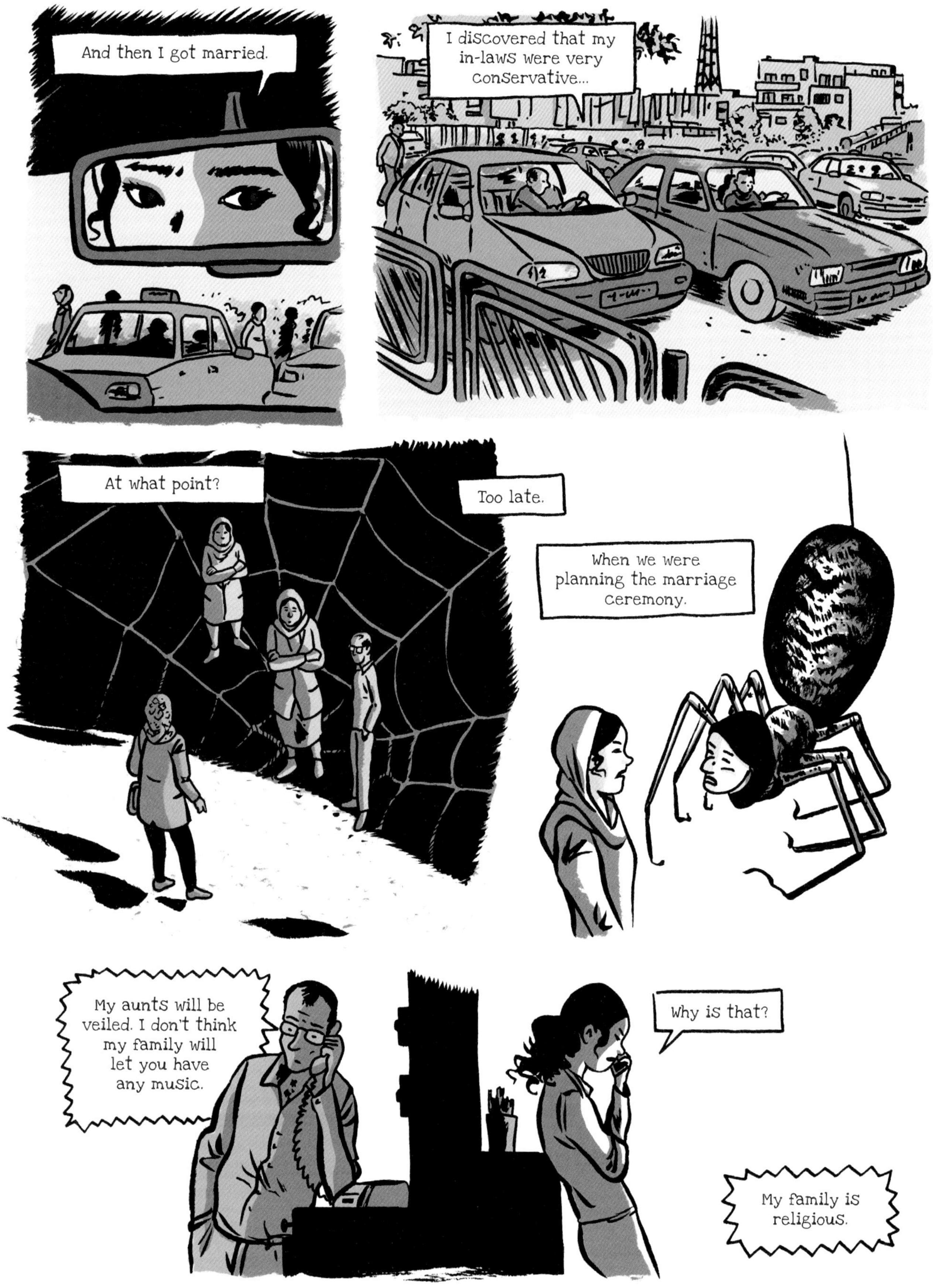
And then I got married.
I discovered that my in-laws were very conservative...
At what point?
Too late.
When we were planning the marriage ceremony.
My aunts will be veiled. I don't think my family will let you have any music.
Why is that?
My family is religious.

I argued with his parents a lot. They wanted separate celebrations, the men in one place and the women in another...

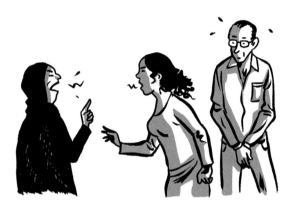

In the end we had a mixed celebration.

But his aunts didn't come.

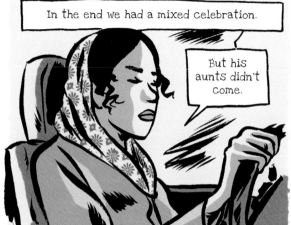

After the wedding, the problems continued. Every time the family got together, it was hell.

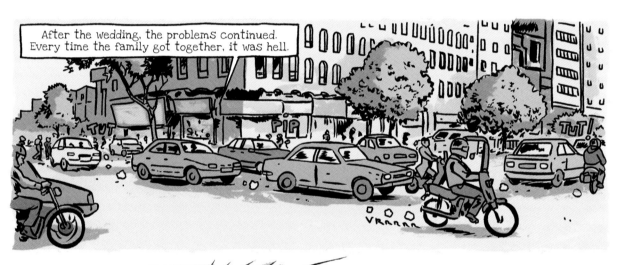

I found out that the women in his family cover themselves— even at home.

I refused to do that...

In the Islamic Republic of Iran, women have to wear the veil in public. They don't need to at home with their family and friends.

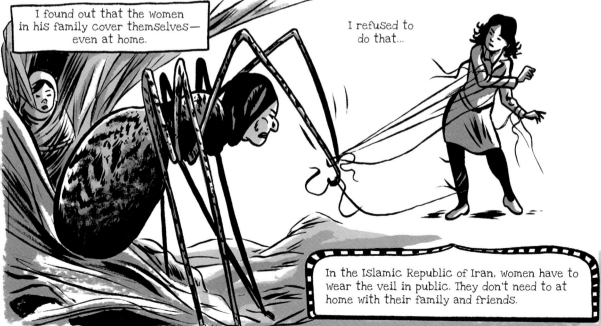

My husband and I started to have terrible arguments.
It went on for 2 years... all of it over the veil.

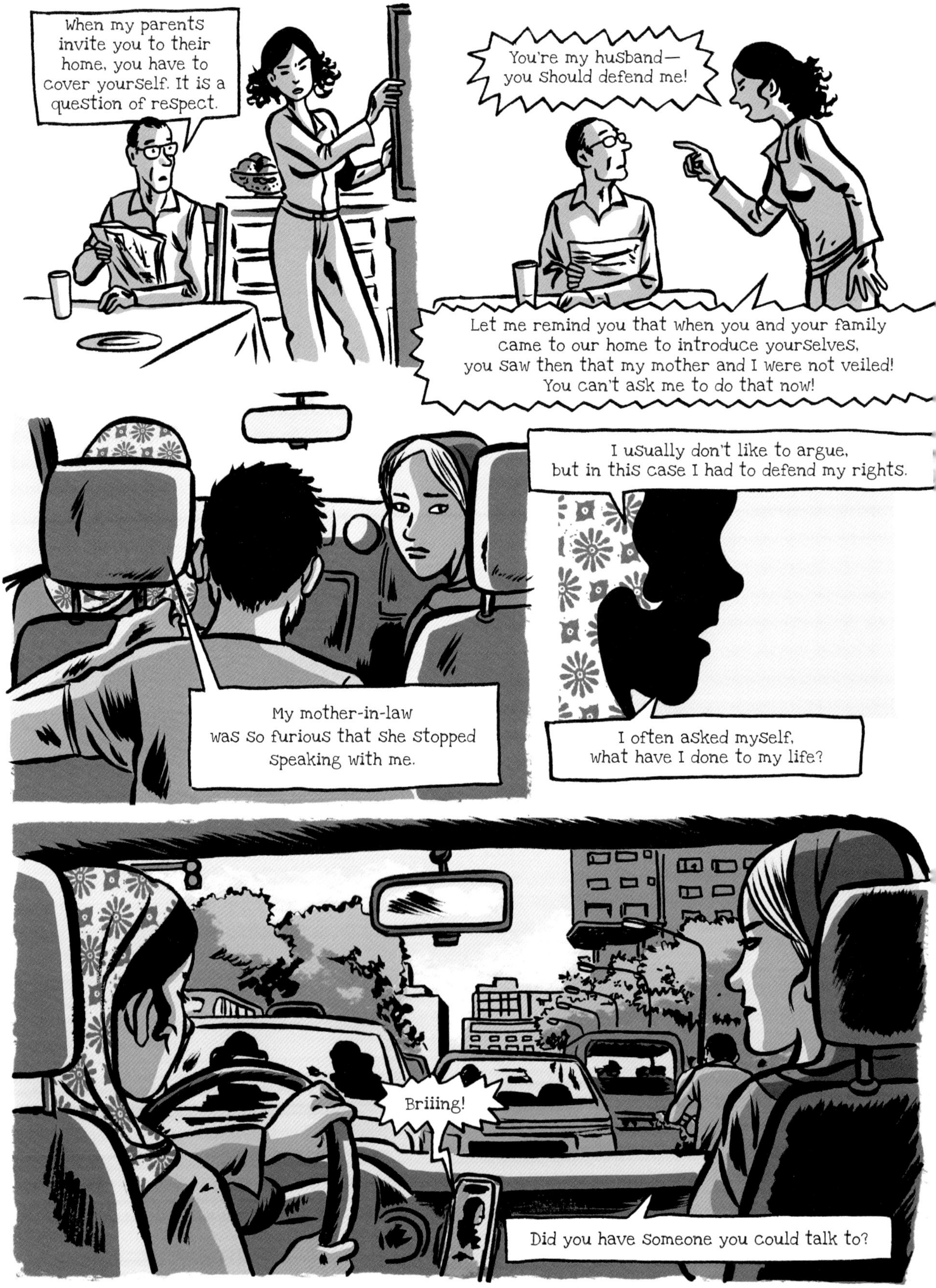

When my parents invite you to their home, you have to cover yourself. It is a question of respect.
You're my husband—you should defend me!
Let me remind you that when you and your family came to our home to introduce yourselves, you saw then that my mother and I were not veiled! You can't ask me to do that now!
I usually don't like to argue, but in this case I had to defend my rights.
My mother-in-law was so furious that she stopped speaking with me.
I often asked myself, what have I done to my life?
Briiing!
Did you have someone you could talk to?

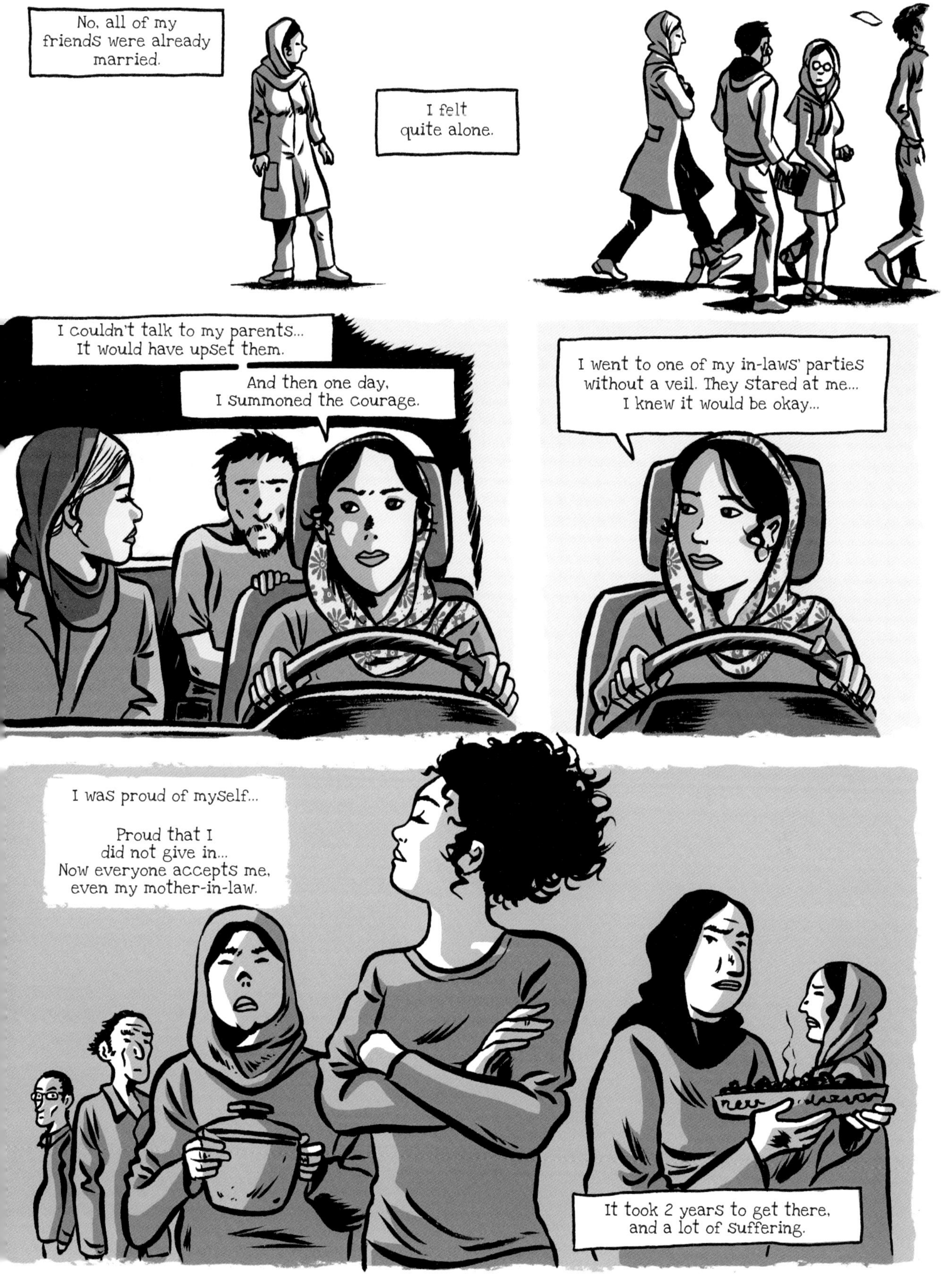
No, all of my friends were already married.
I felt quite alone.
I couldn't talk to my parents... It would have upset them.
And then one day, I summoned the courage.
I went to one of my in-laws' parties without a veil. They stared at me... I knew it would be okay...
I was proud of myself...
Proud that I did not give in... Now everyone accepts me, even my mother-in-law.
It took 2 years to get there, and a lot of suffering.

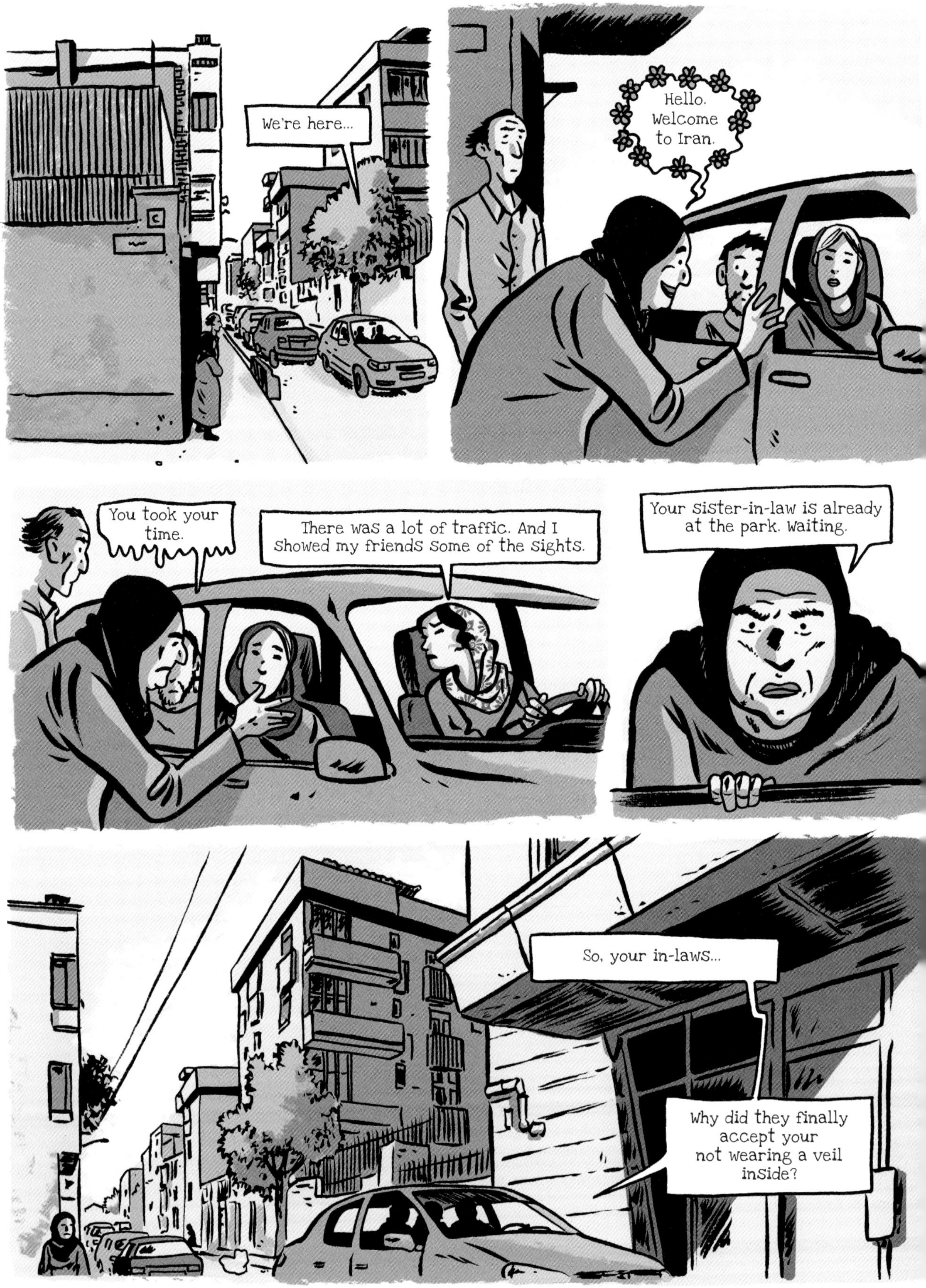
We're here...
Hello. Welcome to Iran.
You took your time.
There was a lot of traffic. And I showed my friends some of the sights.
Your sister-in-law is already at the park. Waiting.
So, your in-laws...
Why did they finally accept your not wearing a veil inside?

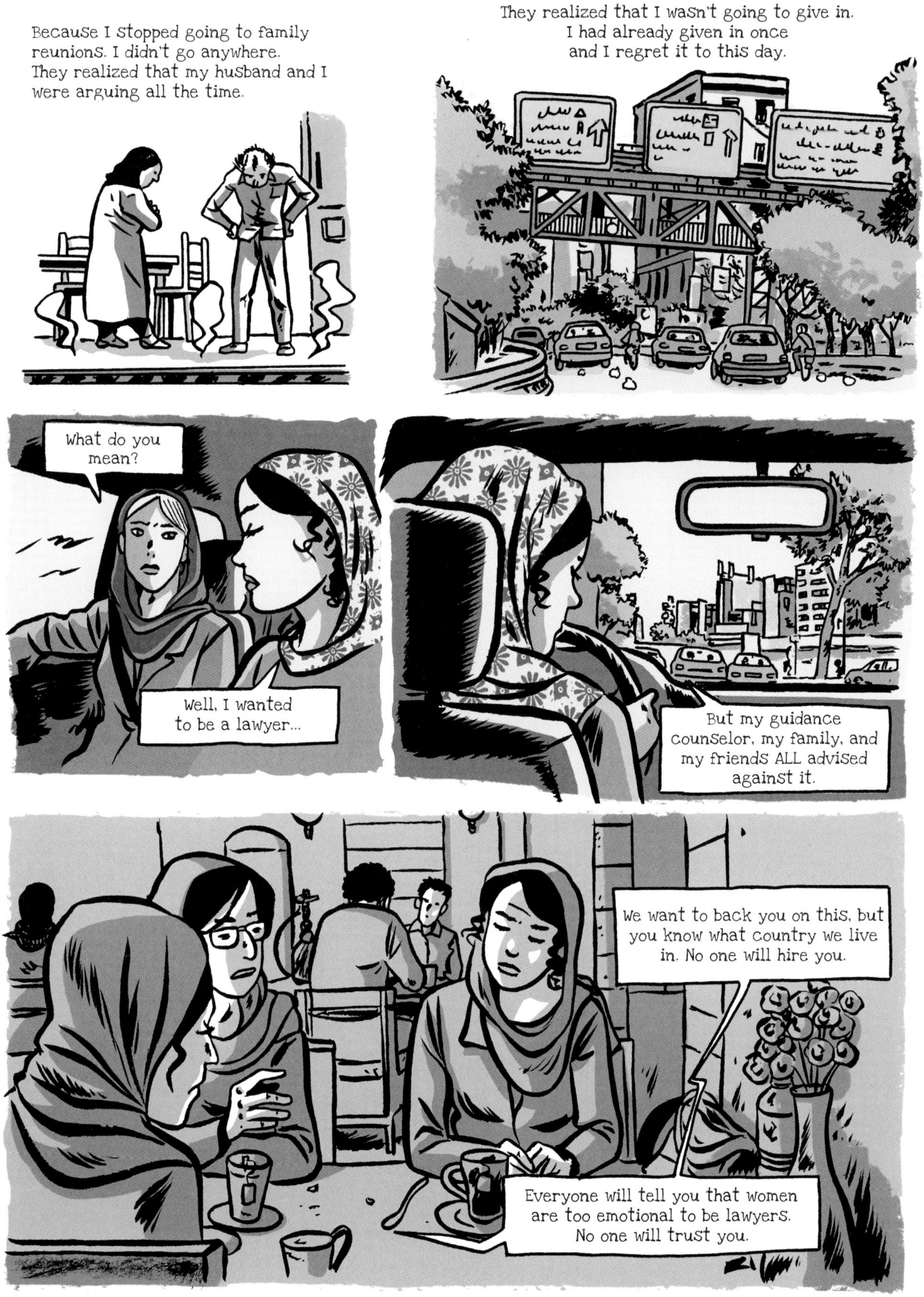
Because I stopped going to family reunions. I didn't go anywhere. They realized that my husband and I were arguing all the time.
They realized that I wasn't going to give in. I had already given in once and I regret it to this day.
What do you mean?
Well, I wanted to be a lawyer...
But my guidance counselor, my family, and my friends ALL advised against it.
We want to back you on this, but you know what country we live in. No one will hire you.
Everyone will tell you that women are too emotional to be lawyers. No one will trust you.

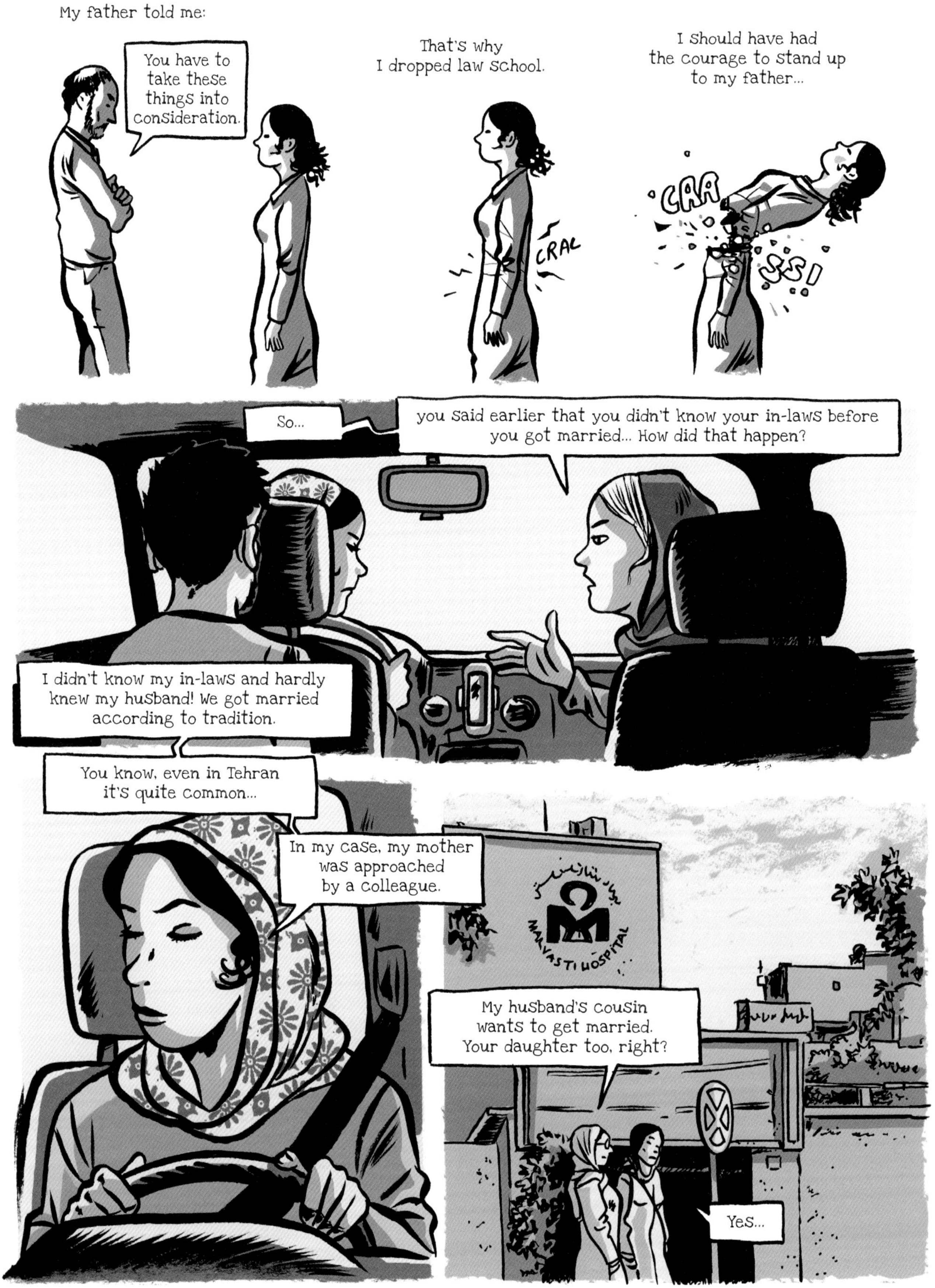
My father told me:
You have to take these things into consideration.
That's why I dropped law school.
CRAC
I should have had the courage to stand up to my father...
CRA
SS!
So...
you said earlier that you didn't know your in-laws before you got married... How did that happen?
I didn't know my in-laws and hardly knew my husband! We got married according to tradition.
You know, even in Tehran it's quite common...
In my case, my mother was approached by a colleague.
MAVASTI HOSPITAL
My husband's cousin wants to get married. Your daughter too, right?
Yes...

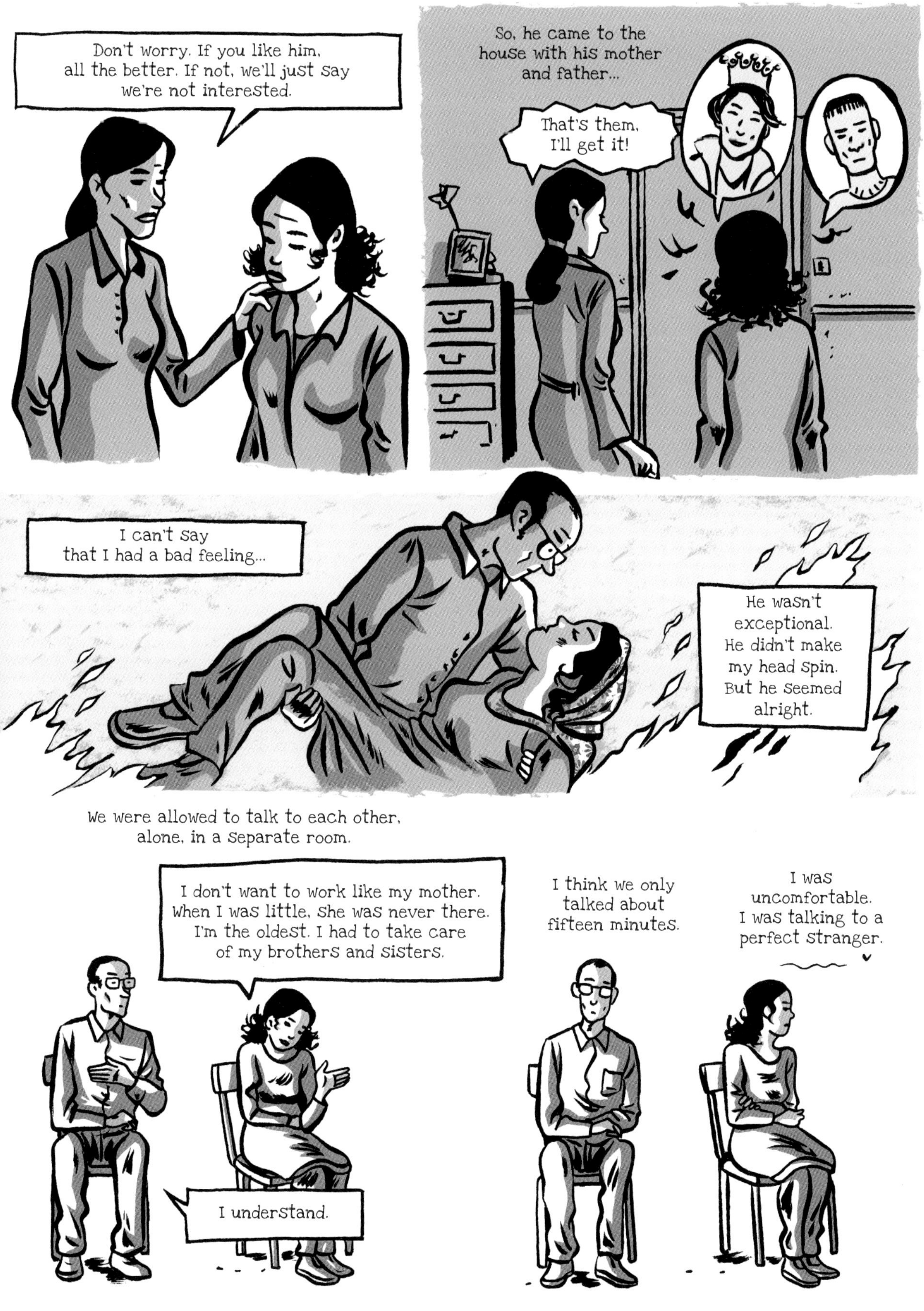
Don't worry. If you like him, all the better. If not, we'll just say we're not interested.
So, he came to the house with his mother and father...
That's them, I'll get it!
I can't say that I had a bad feeling...
He wasn't exceptional. He didn't make my head spin. But he seemed alright.
We were allowed to talk to each other, alone, in a separate room.
I don't want to work like my mother. When I was little, she was never there. I'm the oldest. I had to take care of my brothers and sisters.
I understand.
I think we only talked about fifteen minutes.
I was uncomfortable. I was talking to a perfect stranger.

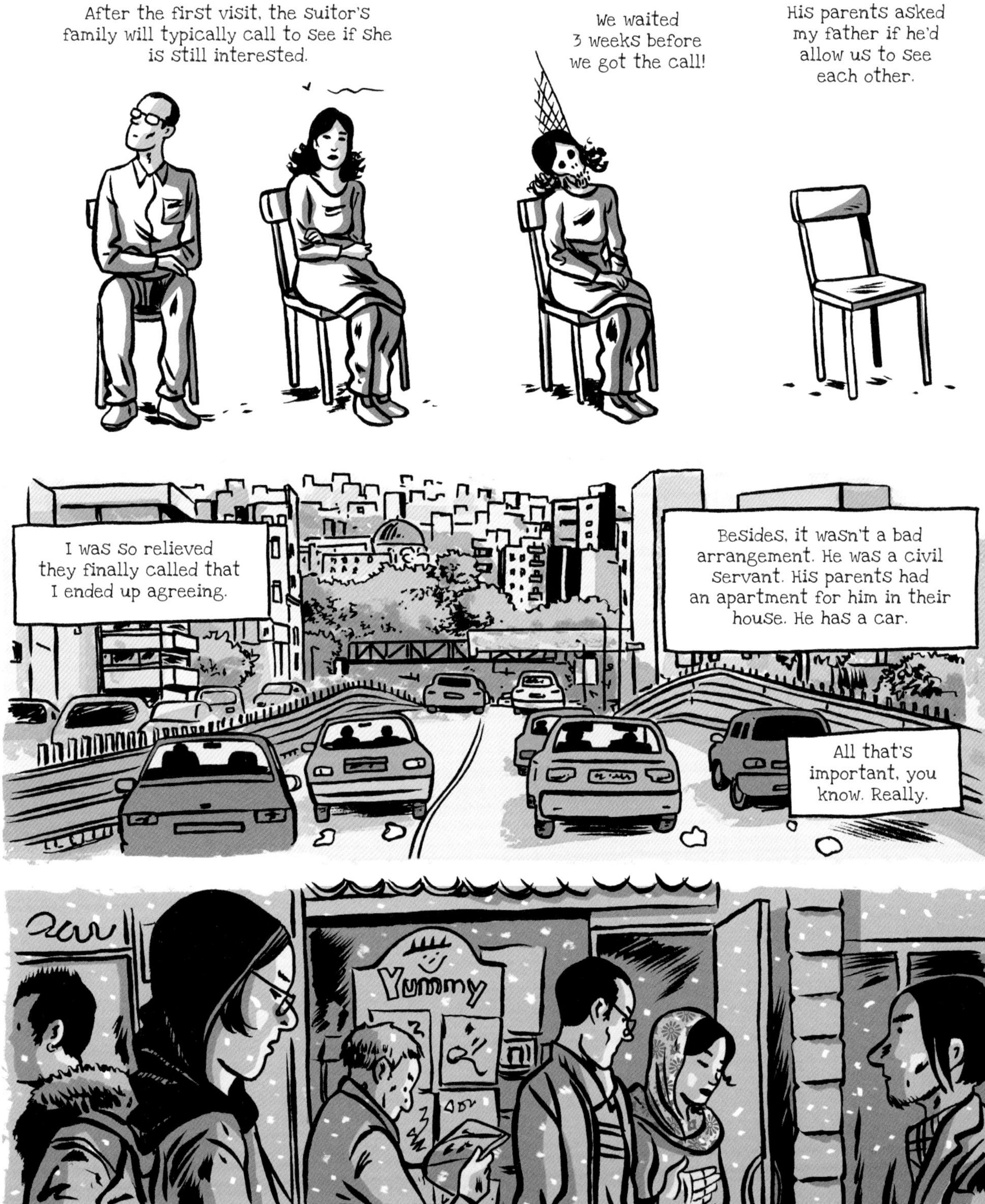
After the first visit, the suitor's family will typically call to see if she is still interested.
We waited 3 weeks before we got the call!
His parents asked my father if he'd allow us to see each other.
I was so relieved they finally called that I ended up agreeing.
Besides, it wasn't a bad arrangement. He was a civil servant. His parents had an apartment for him in their house. He has a car.
All that's important, you know. Really.
Yummy
We started seeing each other. We saw each other every day during the year-end holidays. And when we couldn't see each other we spoke on the phone.
At the end of the month, we told my parents that we were ready to get married.

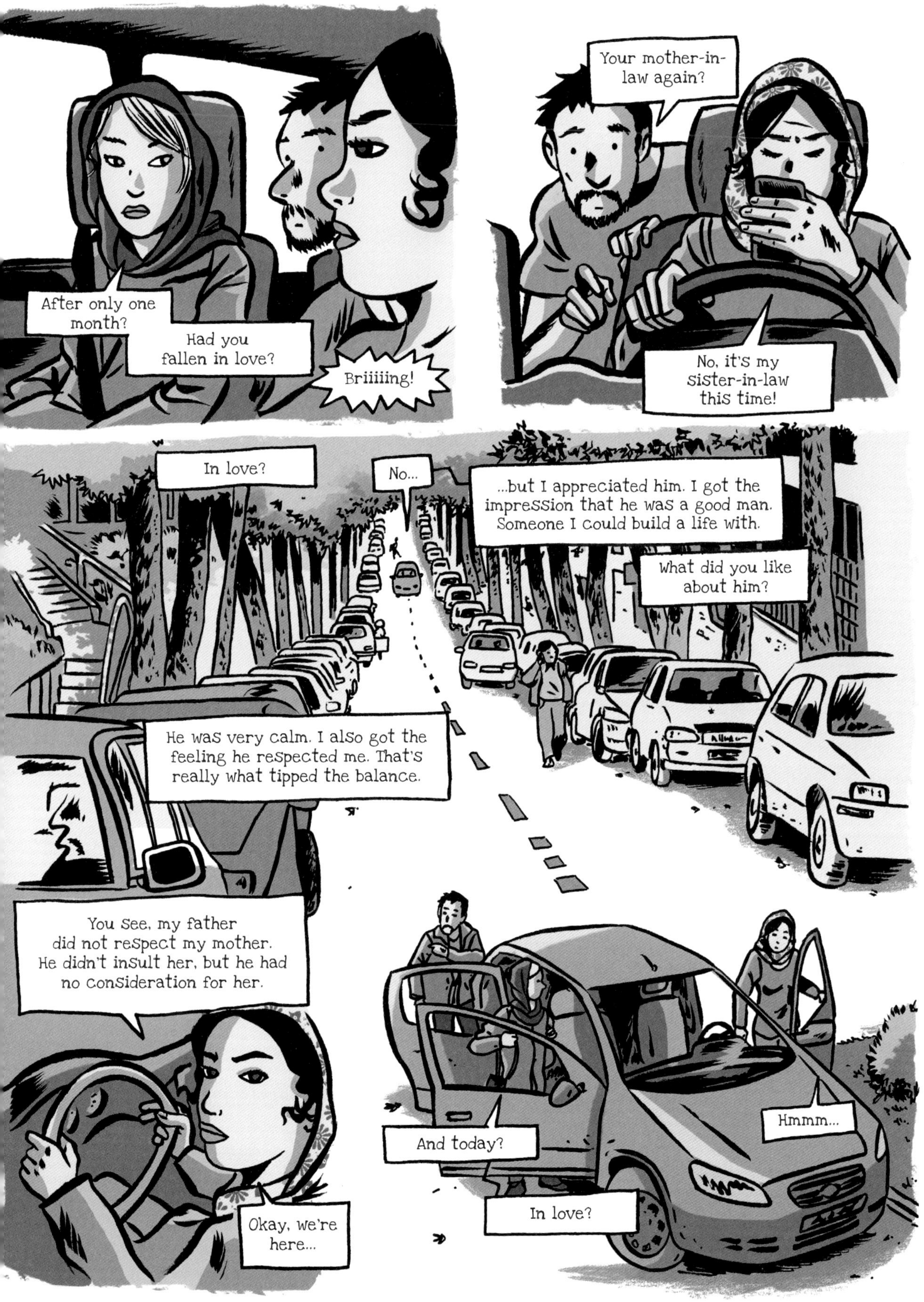

After only one month?
Had you fallen in love?
Briiiing!
Your mother-in-law again?
No, it's my sister-in-law this time!
In love?
No...
...but I appreciated him. I got the impression that he was a good man. Someone I could build a life with.
What did you like about him?
He was very calm. I also got the feeling he respected me. That's really what tipped the balance.
You see, my father did not respect my mother. He didn't insult her, but he had no consideration for her.
Okay, we're here...
And today?
Hmmm...
In love?

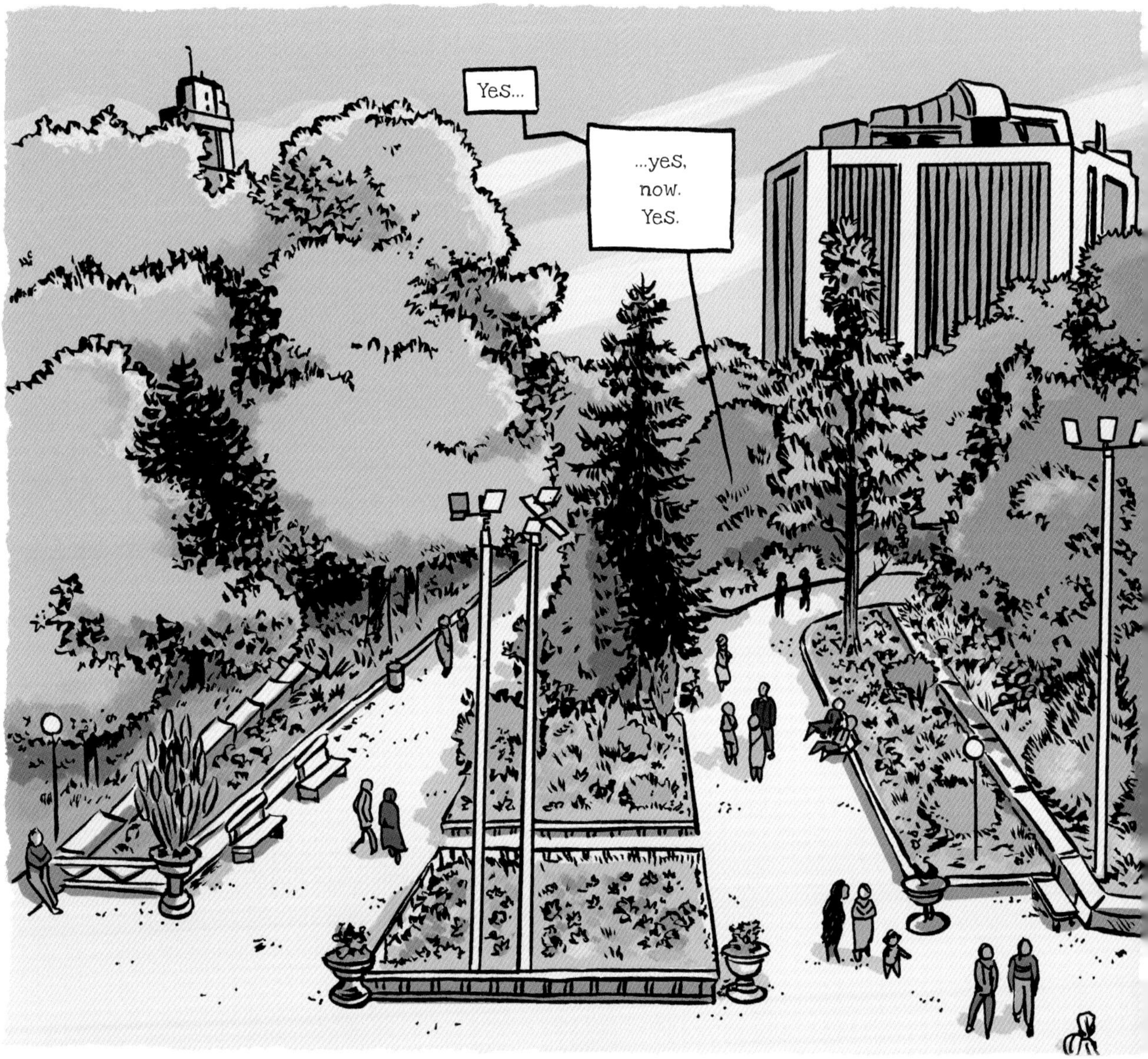
Yes...
...yes,
now.
Yes.

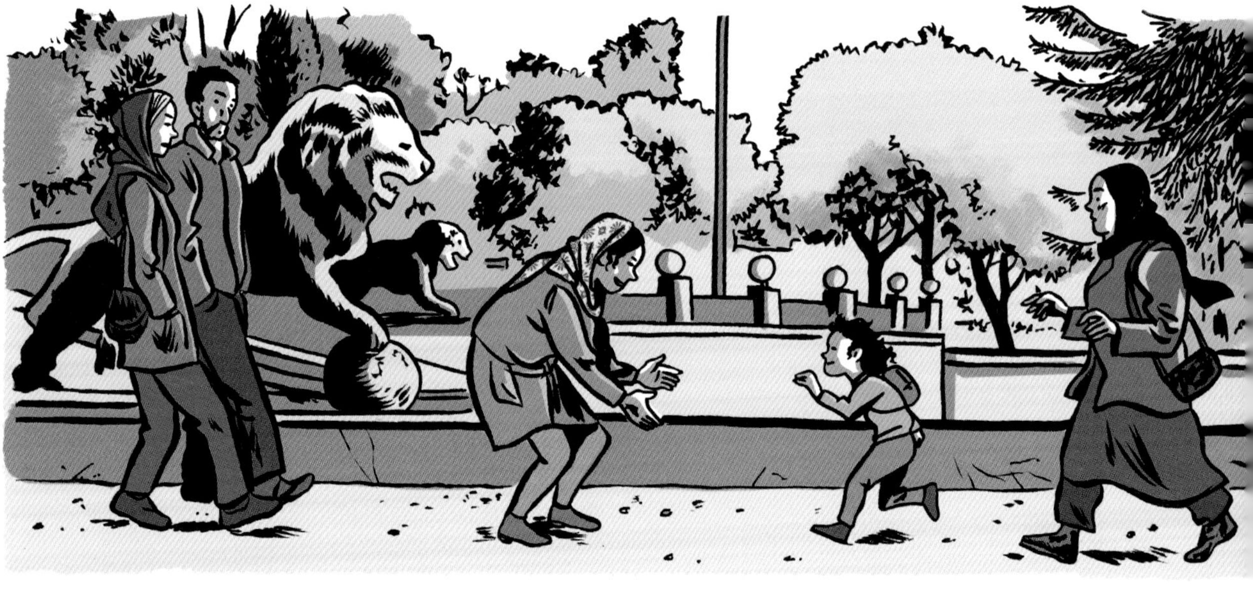

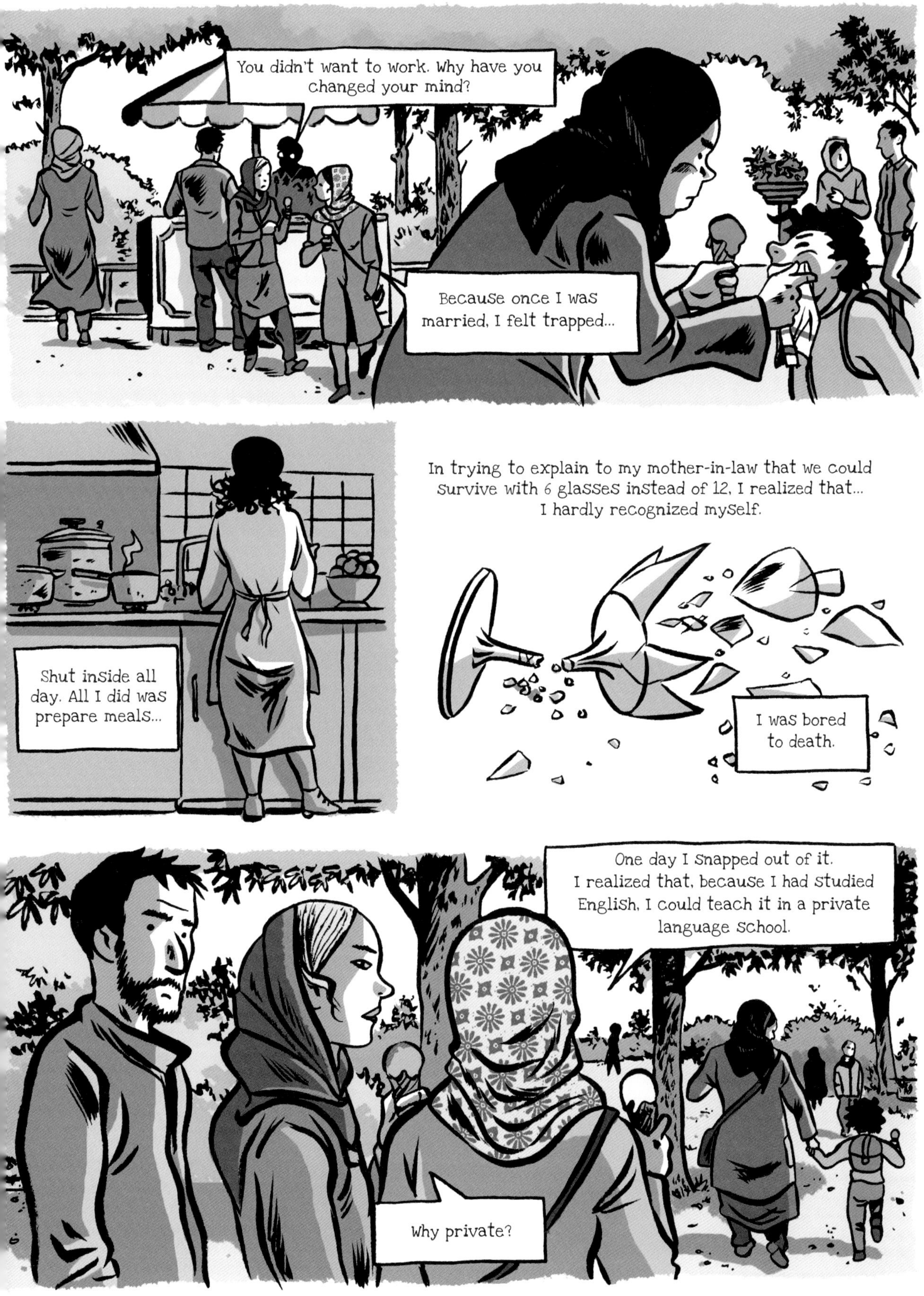
You didn't want to work. Why have you changed your mind?
Because once I was married, I felt trapped...
Shut inside all day. All I did was prepare meals...
In trying to explain to my mother-in-law that we could survive with 6 glasses instead of 12, I realized that... I hardly recognized myself.
I was bored to death.
One day I snapped out of it. I realized that, because I had studied English, I could teach it in a private language school.
Why private?

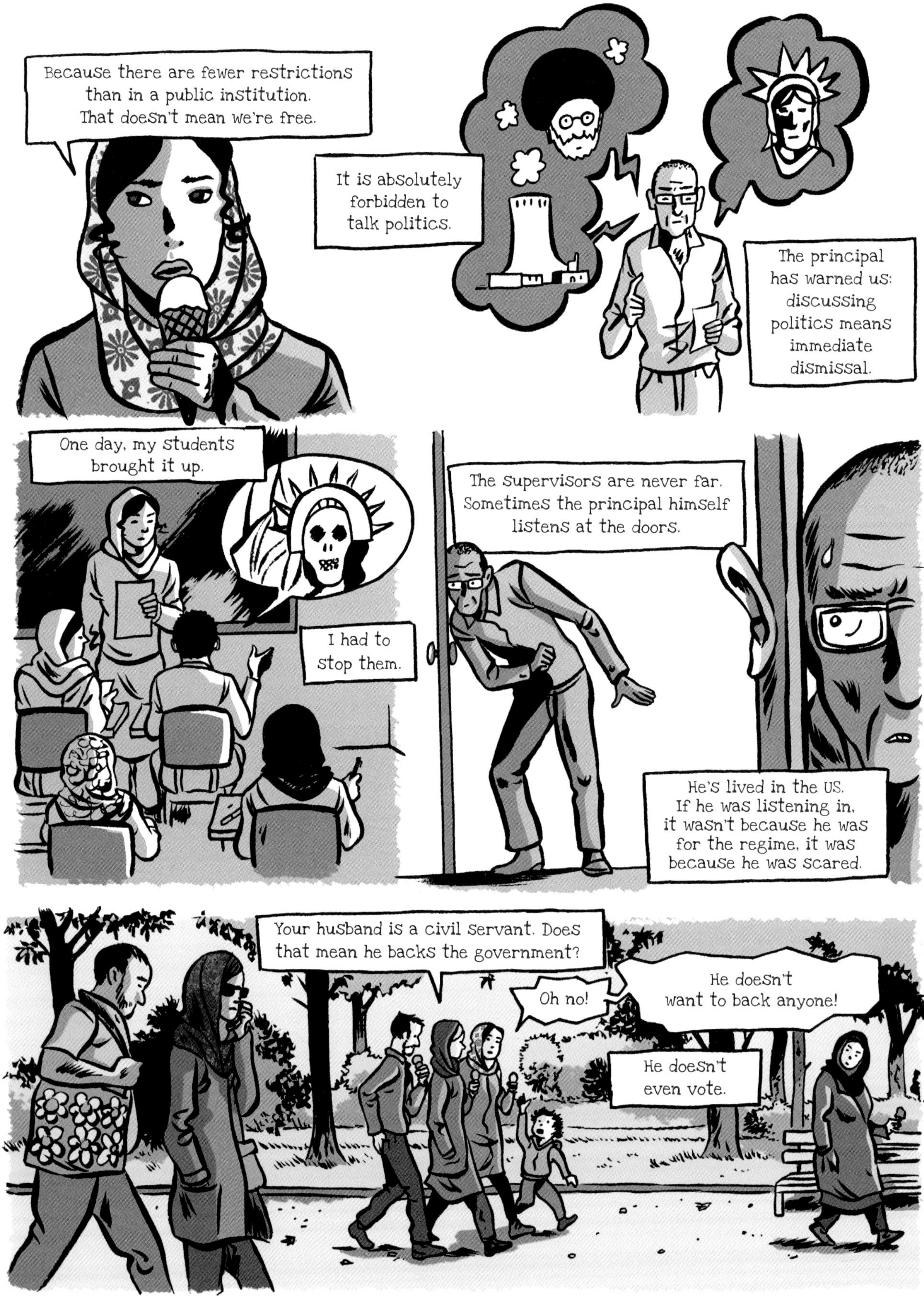

Because there are fewer restrictions than in a public institution. That doesn't mean we're free.
It is absolutely forbidden to talk politics.
The principal has warned us: discussing politics means immediate dismissal.
One day, my students brought it up.
I had to stop them.
The supervisors are never far. Sometimes the principal himself listens at the doors.
He's lived in the US. If he was listening in, it wasn't because he was for the regime, it was because he was scared.
Your husband is a civil servant. Does that mean he backs the government?
Oh no!
He doesn't want to back anyone!
He doesn't even vote.

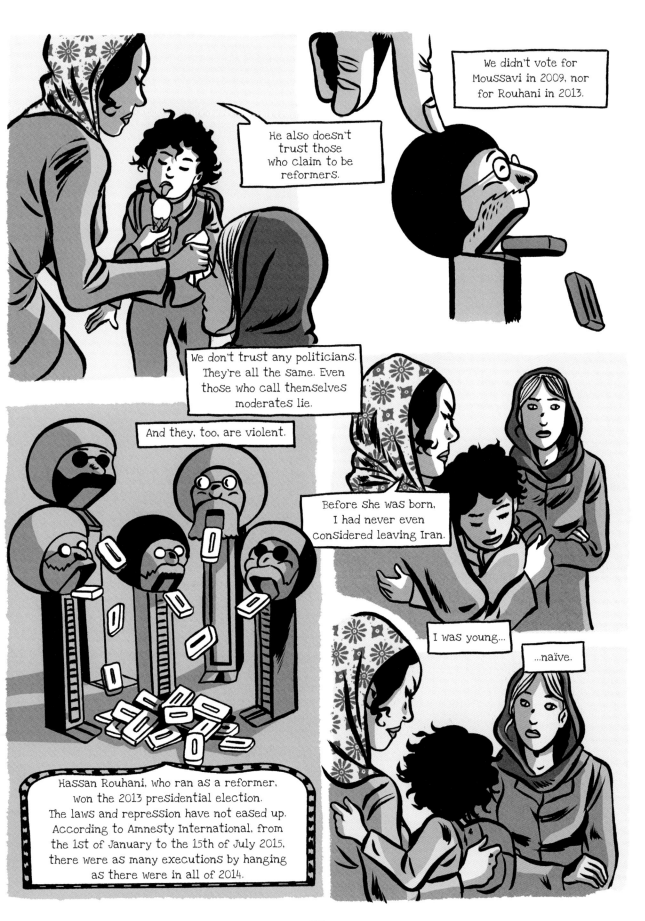

He also doesn't trust those who claim to be reformers.

We didn't vote for Moussavi in 2009, nor for Rouhani in 2013.

We don't trust any politicians. They're all the same. Even those who call themselves moderates lie.

And they, too, are violent.

Before she was born, I had never even considered leaving Iran.

Hassan Rouhani, who ran as a reformer, won the 2013 presidential election. The laws and repression have not eased up. According to Amnesty International, from the 1st of January to the 15th of July 2015, there were as many executions by hanging as there were in all of 2014.

I was young...

...naïve.

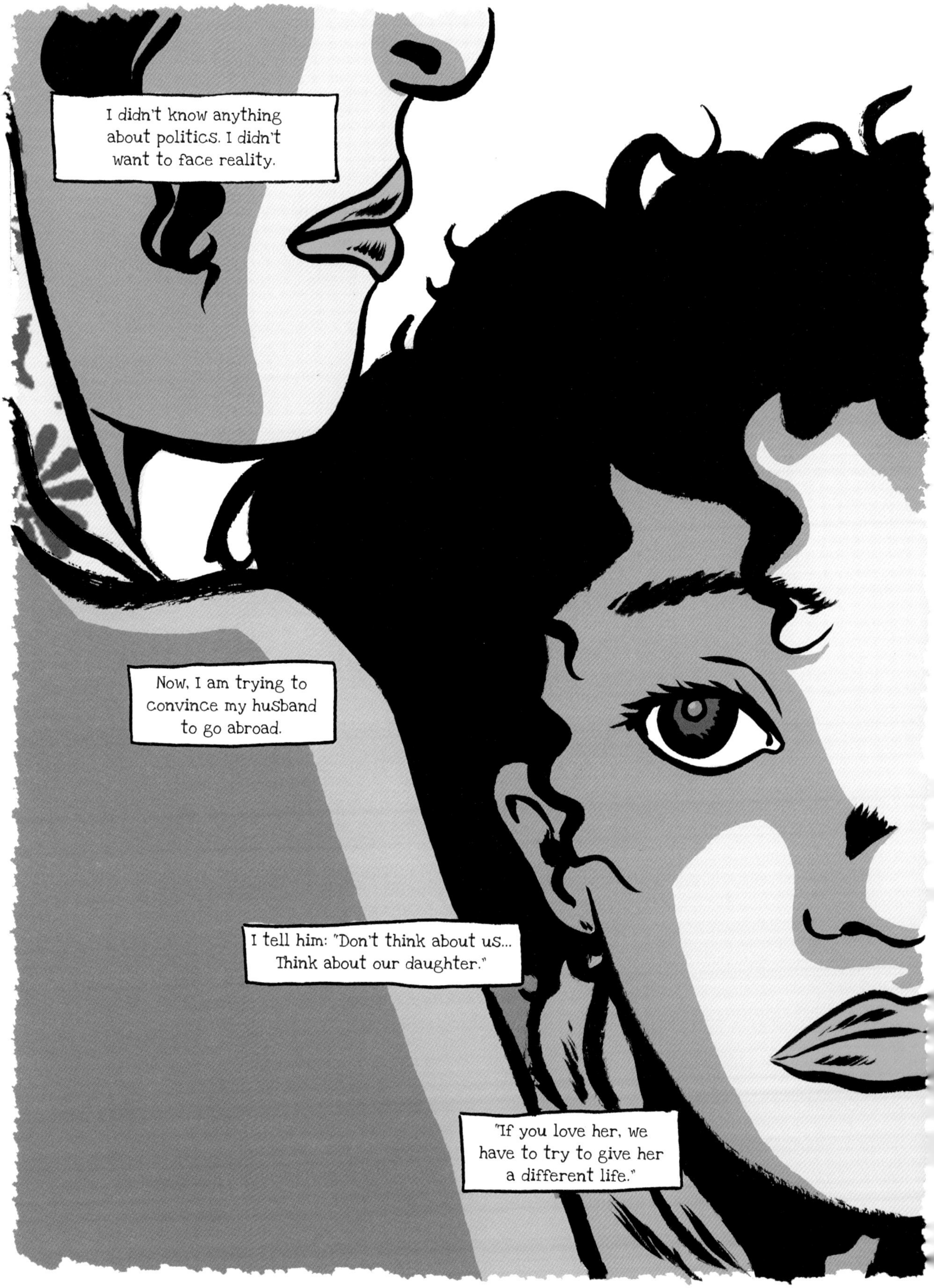
I didn't know anything about politics. I didn't want to face reality.
Now, I am trying to convince my husband to go abroad.
I tell him: "Don't think about us... Think about our daughter."
"If you love her, we have to try to give her a different life."

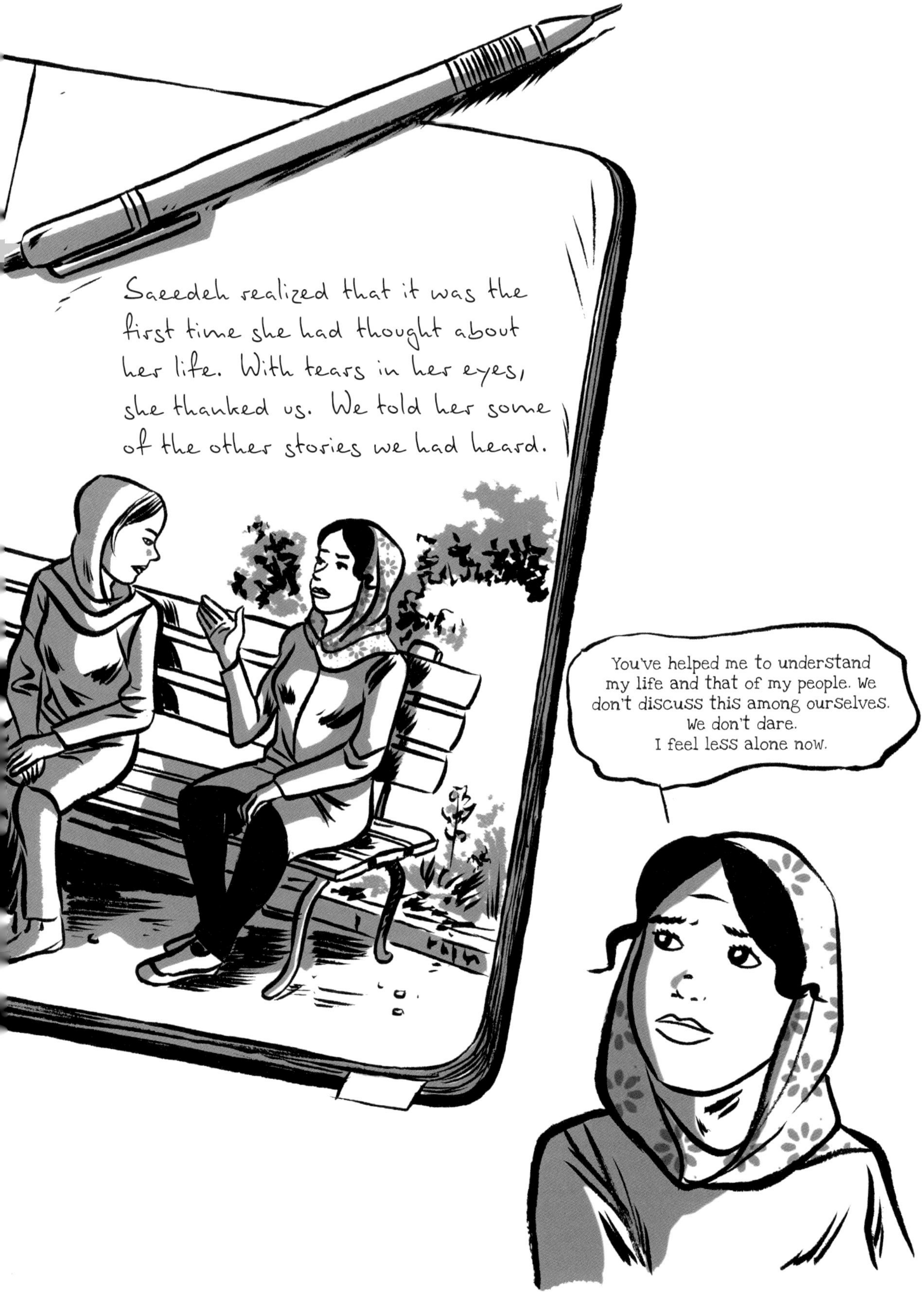
Saeedeh realized that it was the first time she had thought about her life. With tears in her eyes, she thanked us. We told her some of the other stories we had heard.
You've helped me to understand my life and that of my people. We don't discuss this among ourselves. We don't dare. I feel less alone now.

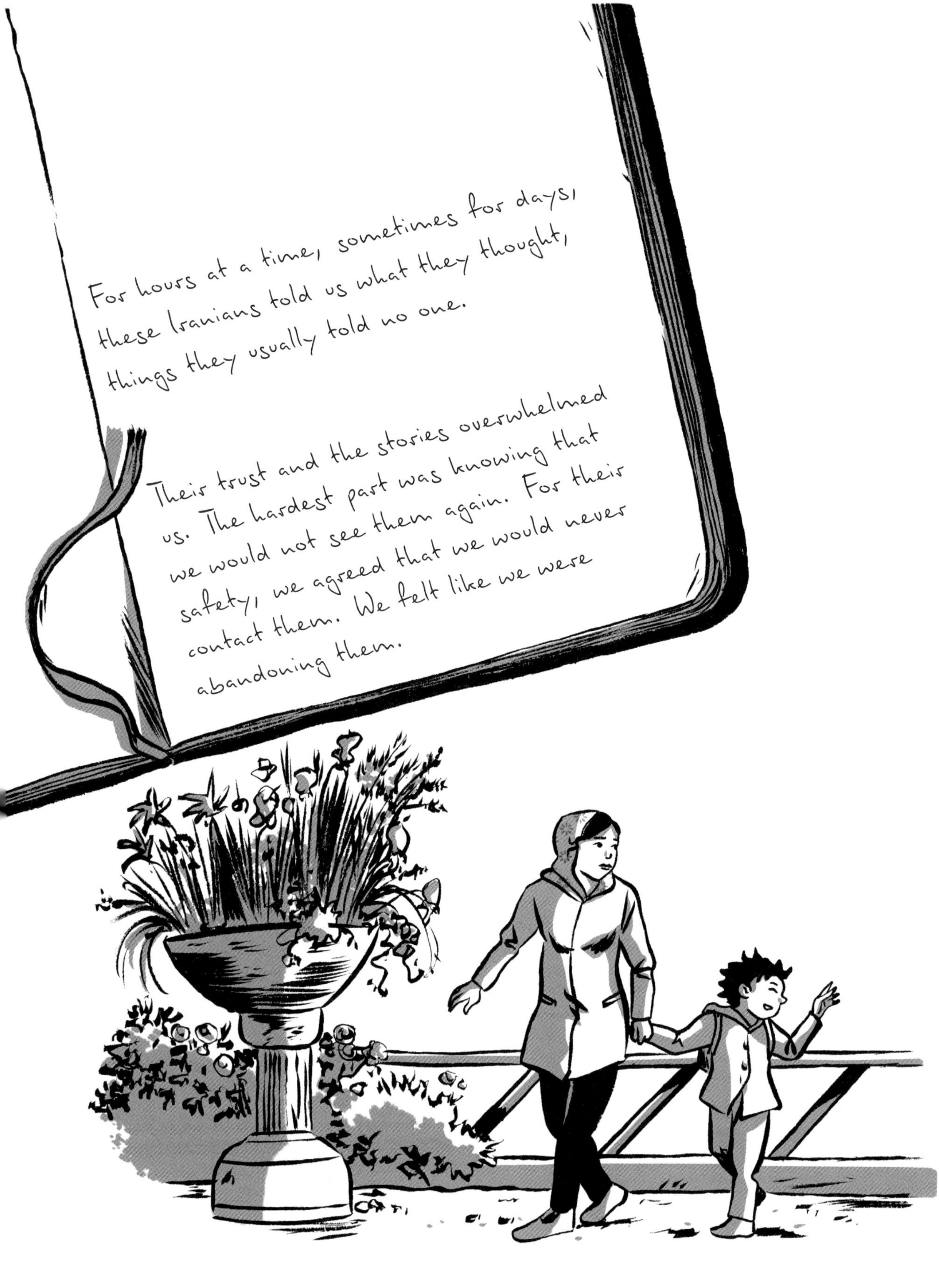
For hours at a time, sometimes for days, these Iranians told us what they thought, things they usually told no one.
Their trust and the stories overwhelmed us. The hardest part was knowing that we would not see them again. For their safety, we agreed that we would never contact them. We felt like we were abandoning them.

SOBAN, 28,
Mashhad.

Soban had everything you
need to have a great life.
He wanted to share it with the
woman he loved.

A closet romantic at heart.

His wife would be selected
in the traditional way,
not by him.

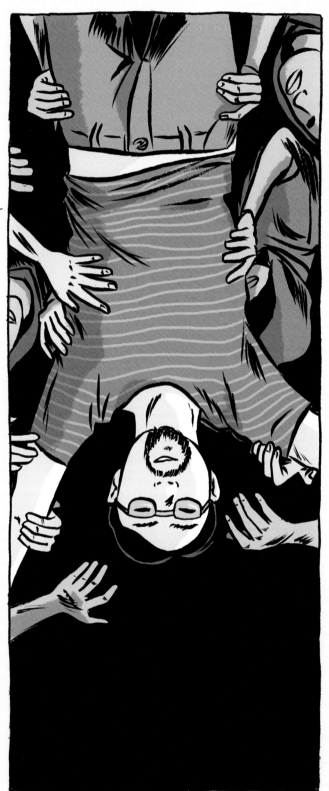

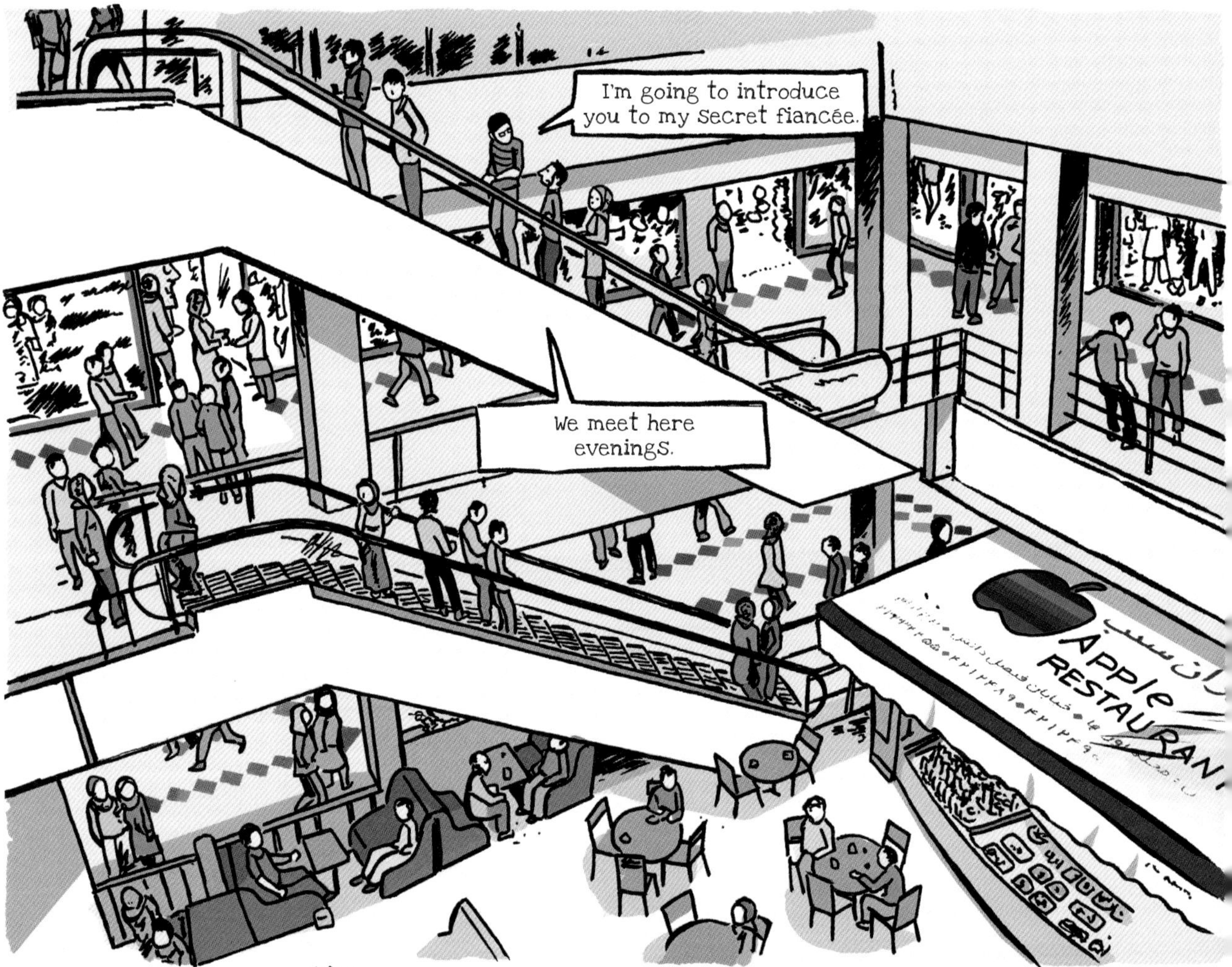
I'm going to introduce you to my secret fiancée.
We meet here evenings.
Apple
RESTAURANT

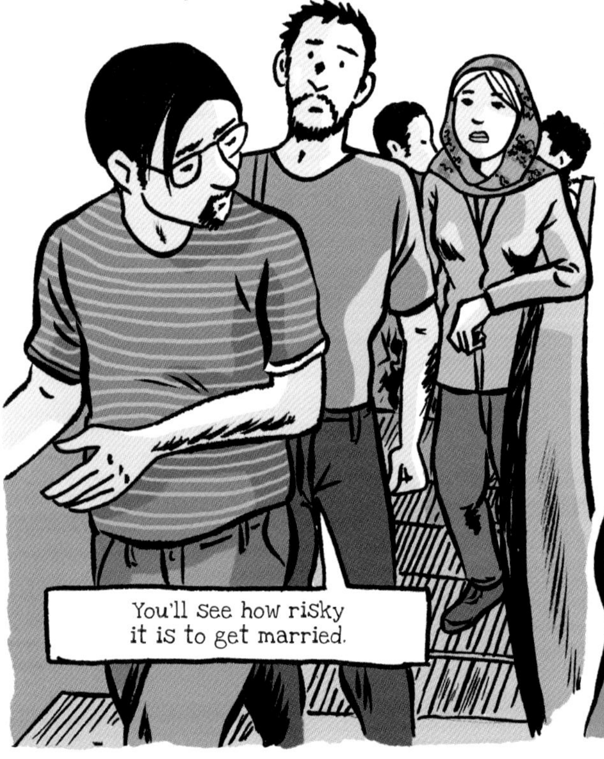
You'll see how risky it is to get married.

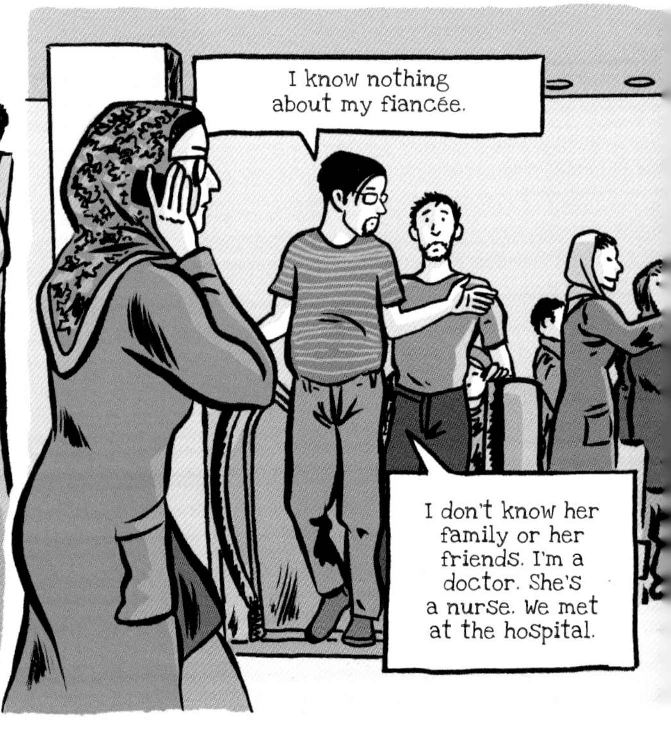
I know nothing about my fiancée.
I don't know her family or her friends. I'm a doctor. She's a nurse. We met at the hospital.

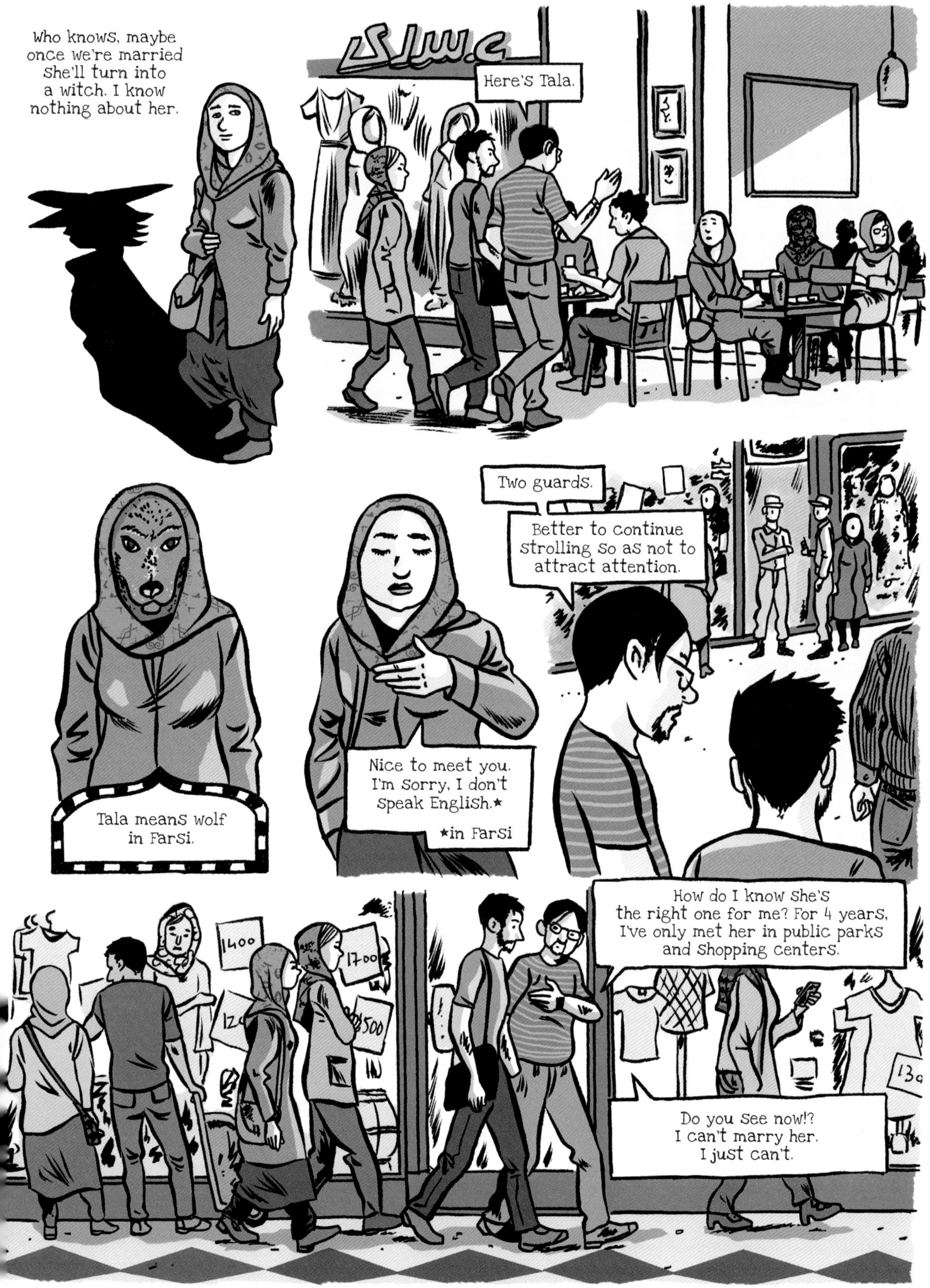

Who knows, maybe once we're married she'll turn into a witch. I know nothing about her.
Here's Tala.
Tala means wolf in Farsi.
Nice to meet you. I'm sorry, I don't speak English.★
★in Farsi
Two guards.
Better to continue strolling so as not to attract attention.
How do I know she's the right one for me? For 4 years, I've only met her in public parks and shopping centers.
Do you see now!? I can't marry her. I just can't.

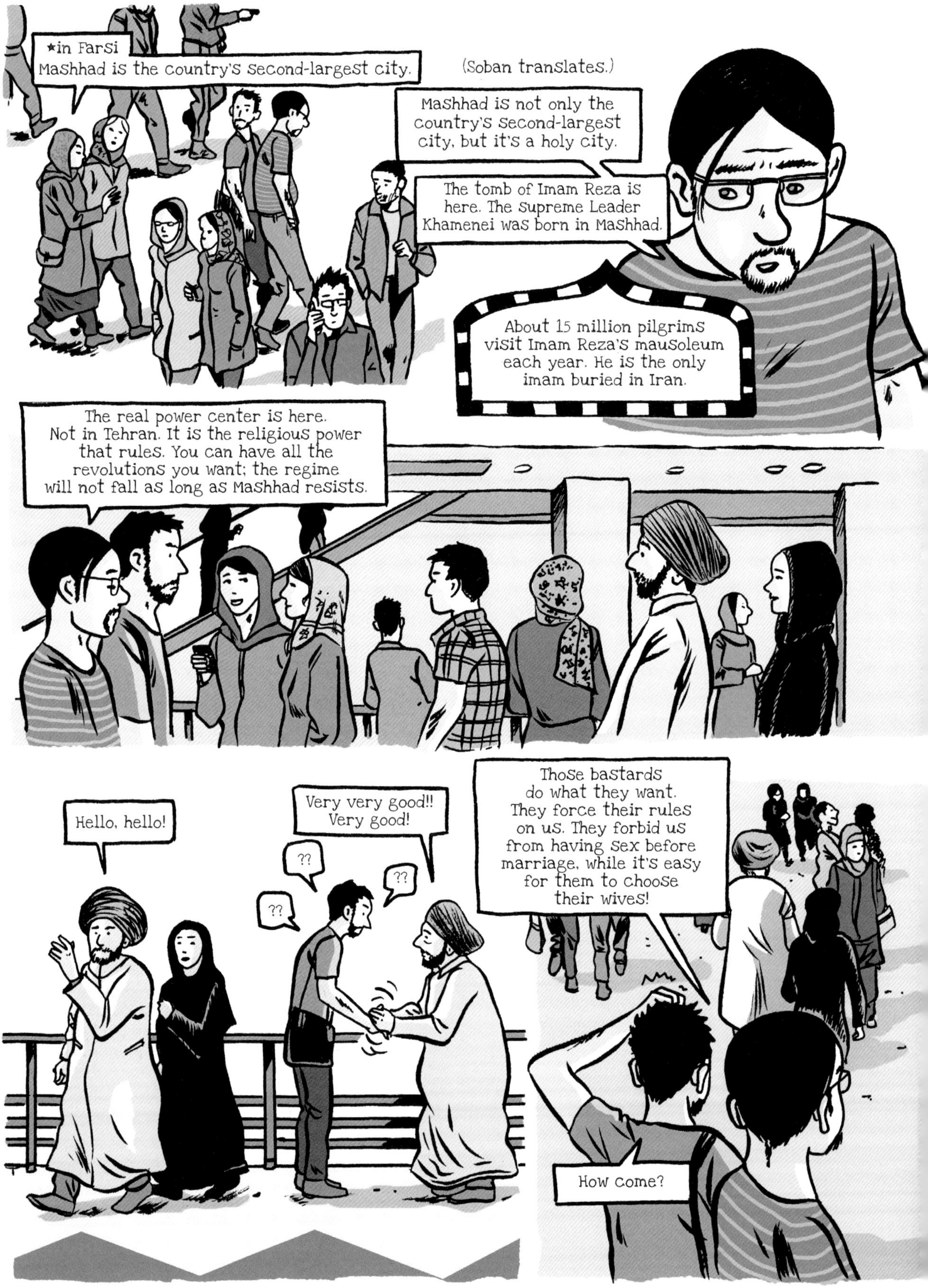
*in Farsi
Mashhad is the country's second-largest city.
(Soban translates.)
Mashhad is not only the country's second-largest city, but it's a holy city.
The tomb of Imam Reza is here. The Supreme Leader Khamenei was born in Mashhad.
About 15 million pilgrims visit Imam Reza's mausoleum each year. He is the only imam buried in Iran.
The real power center is here. Not in Tehran. It is the religious power that rules. You can have all the revolutions you want; the regime will not fall as long as Mashhad resists.
Hello, hello!
Very very good!! Very good!
??
??
??
Those bastards do what they want. They force their rules on us. They forbid us from having sex before marriage, while it's easy for them to choose their wives!
How come?

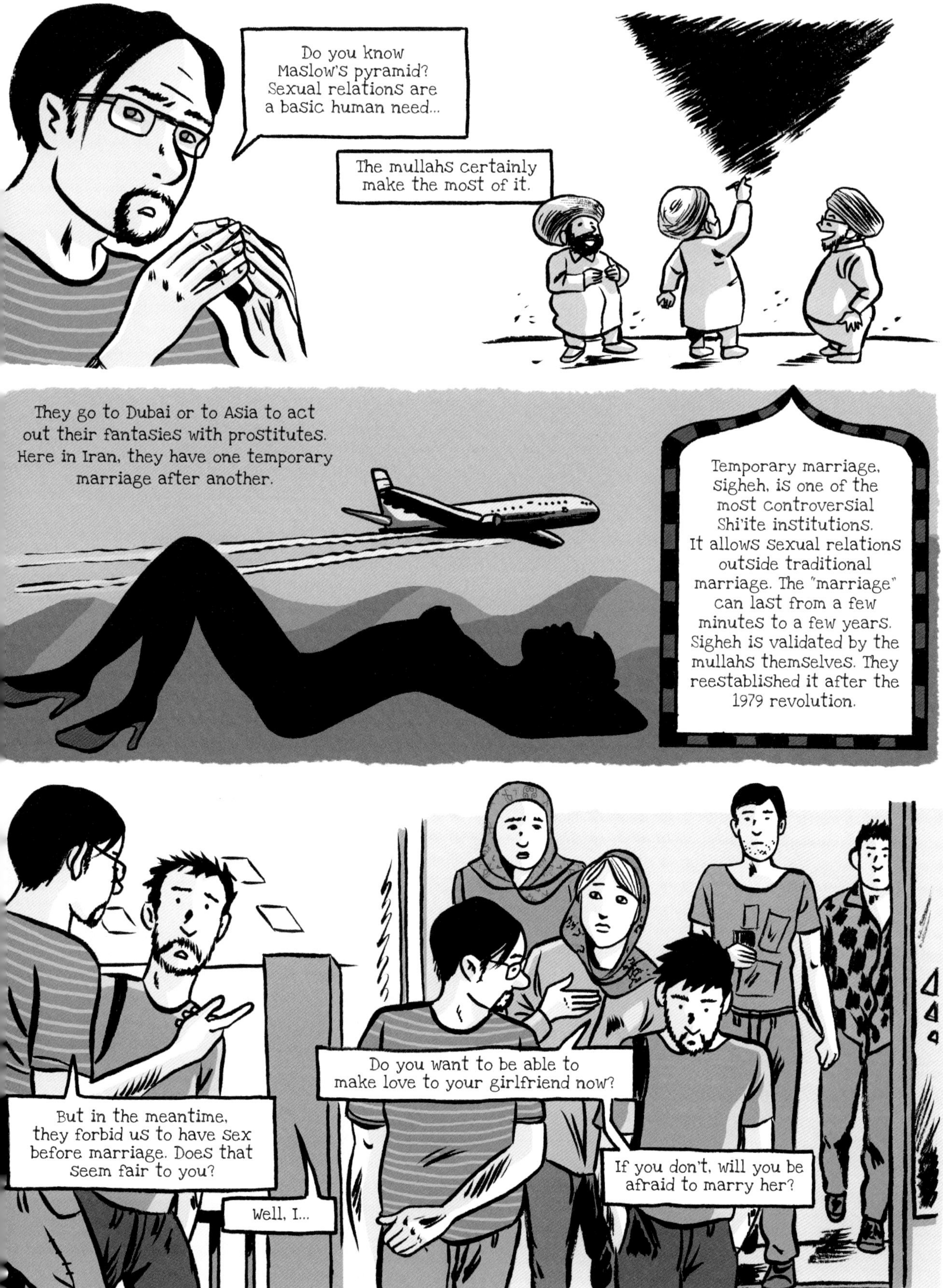
Do you know Maslow's pyramid? Sexual relations are a basic human need...
The mullahs certainly make the most of it.
They go to Dubai or to Asia to act out their fantasies with prostitutes. Here in Iran, they have one temporary marriage after another.
Temporary marriage, sigheh, is one of the most controversial Shi'ite institutions. It allows sexual relations outside traditional marriage. The "marriage" can last from a few minutes to a few years. Sigheh is validated by the mullahs themselves. They reestablished it after the 1979 revolution.
But in the meantime, they forbid us to have sex before marriage. Does that seem fair to you?
Well, I...
Do you want to be able to make love to your girlfriend now?
If you don't, will you be afraid to marry her?

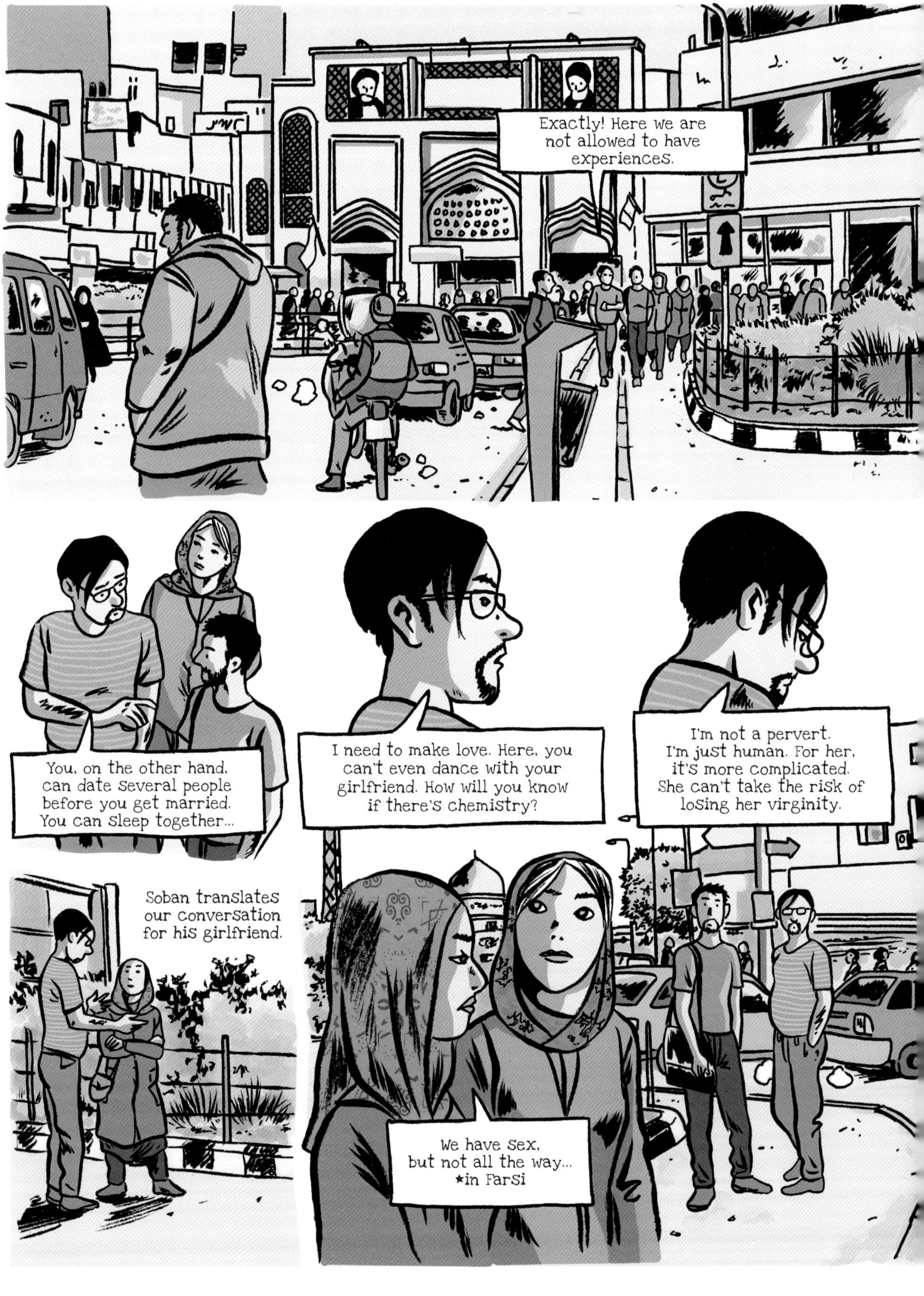
Exactly! Here we are not allowed to have experiences.
You, on the other hand, can date several people before you get married. You can sleep together...
I need to make love. Here, you can't even dance with your girlfriend. How will you know if there's chemistry?
I'm not a pervert. I'm just human. For her, it's more complicated. She can't take the risk of losing her virginity.
Soban translates our conversation for his girlfriend.
We have sex, but not all the way...
*in Farsi

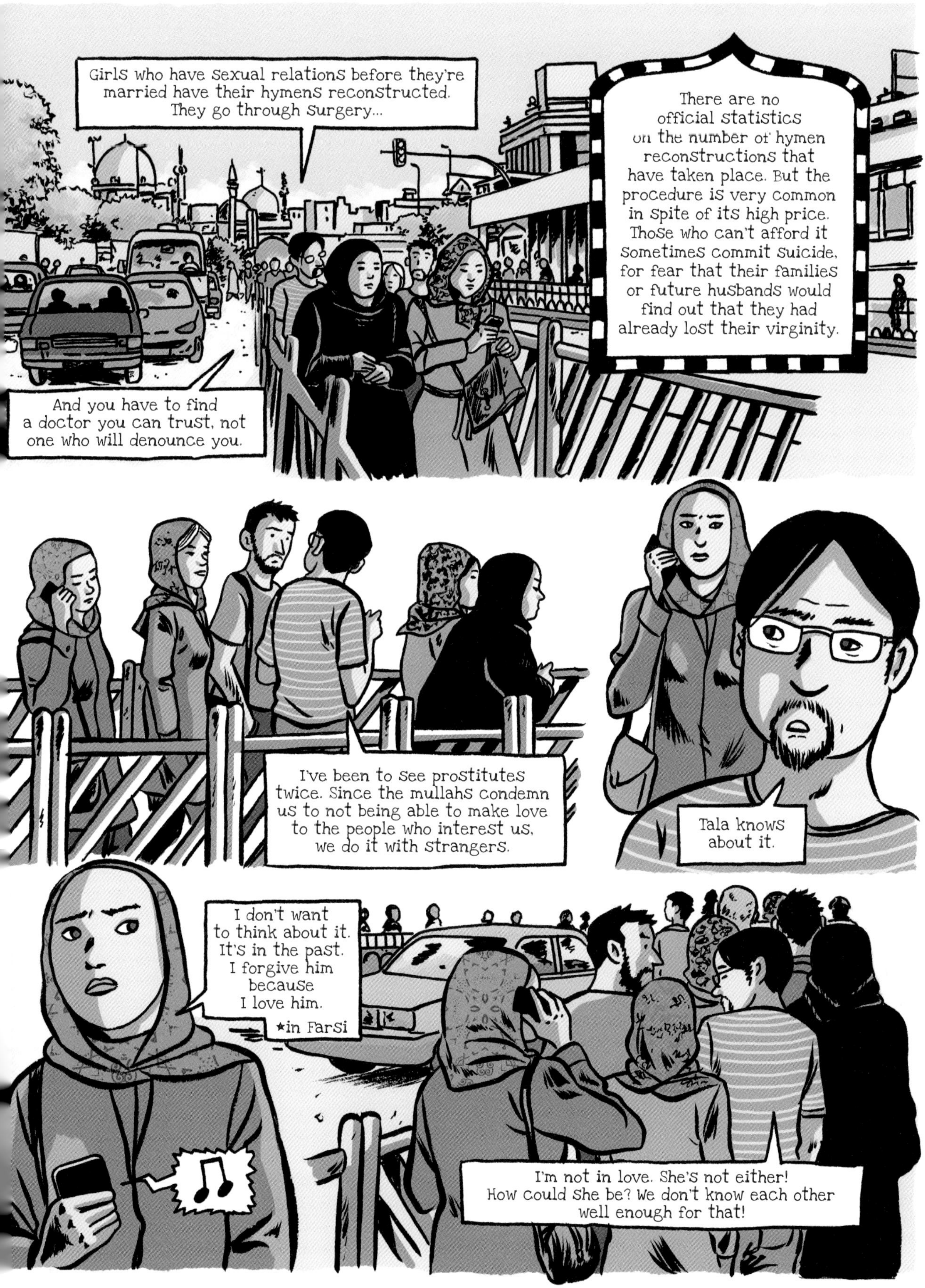
Girls who have sexual relations before they're married have their hymens reconstructed. They go through surgery...
There are no official statistics on the number of hymen reconstructions that have taken place. But the procedure is very common in spite of its high price. Those who can't afford it sometimes commit suicide, for fear that their families or future husbands would find out that they had already lost their virginity.
And you have to find a doctor you can trust, not one who will denounce you.
I've been to see prostitutes twice. Since the mullahs condemn us to not being able to make love to the people who interest us, we do it with strangers.
Tala knows about it.
I don't want to think about it. It's in the past. I forgive him because I love him.
*in Farsi
I'm not in love. She's not either! How could she be? We don't know each other well enough for that!

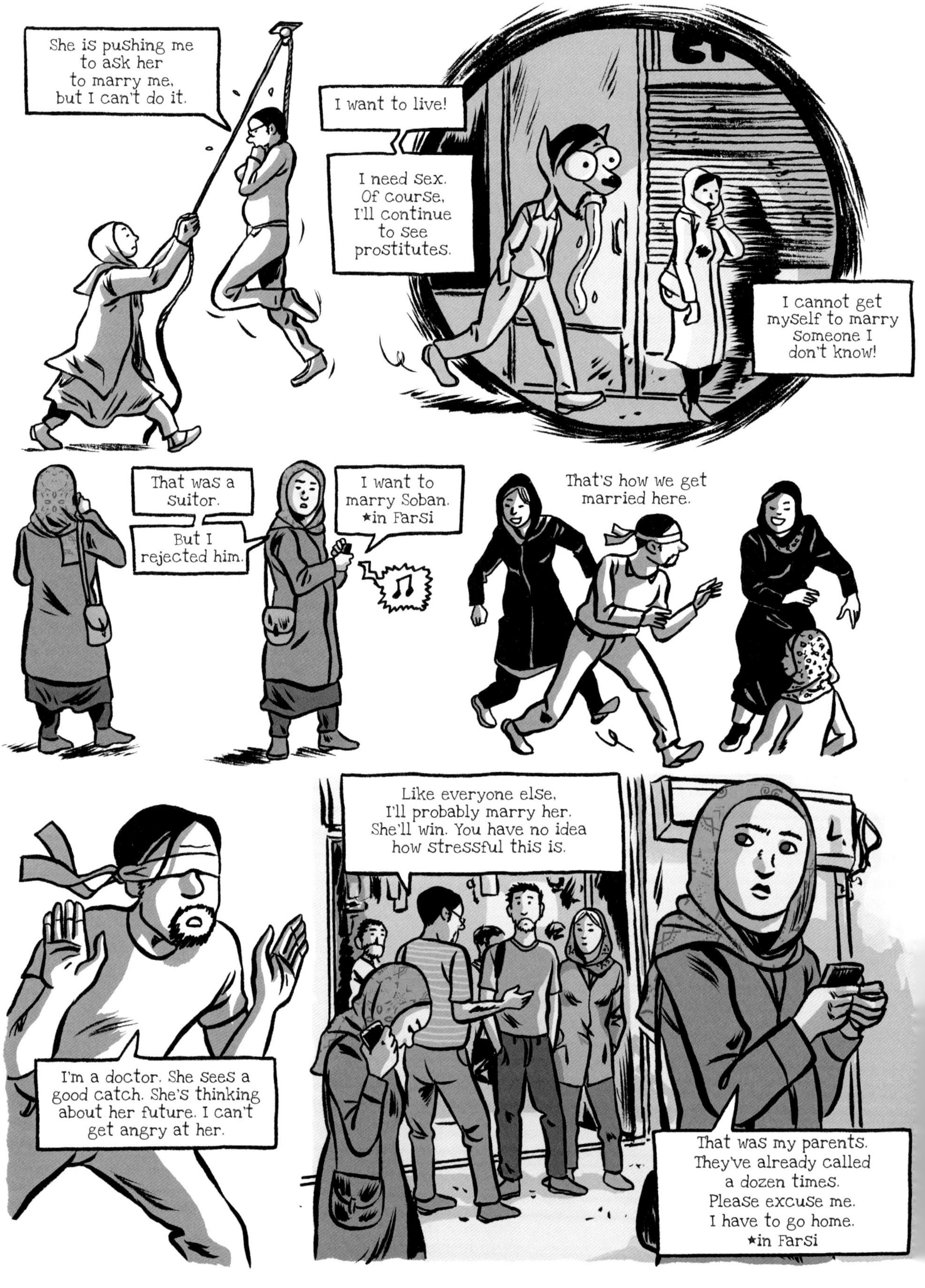

She is pushing me to ask her to marry me, but I can't do it.
I want to live!
I need sex. Of course, I'll continue to see prostitutes.
I cannot get myself to marry someone I don't know!
That was a suitor.
But I rejected him.
I want to marry Soban.
*in Farsi
That's how we get married here.
I'm a doctor. She sees a good catch. She's thinking about her future. I can't get angry at her.
Like everyone else, I'll probably marry her. She'll win. You have no idea how stressful this is.
That was my parents. They've already called a dozen times. Please excuse me. I have to go home.
*in Farsi

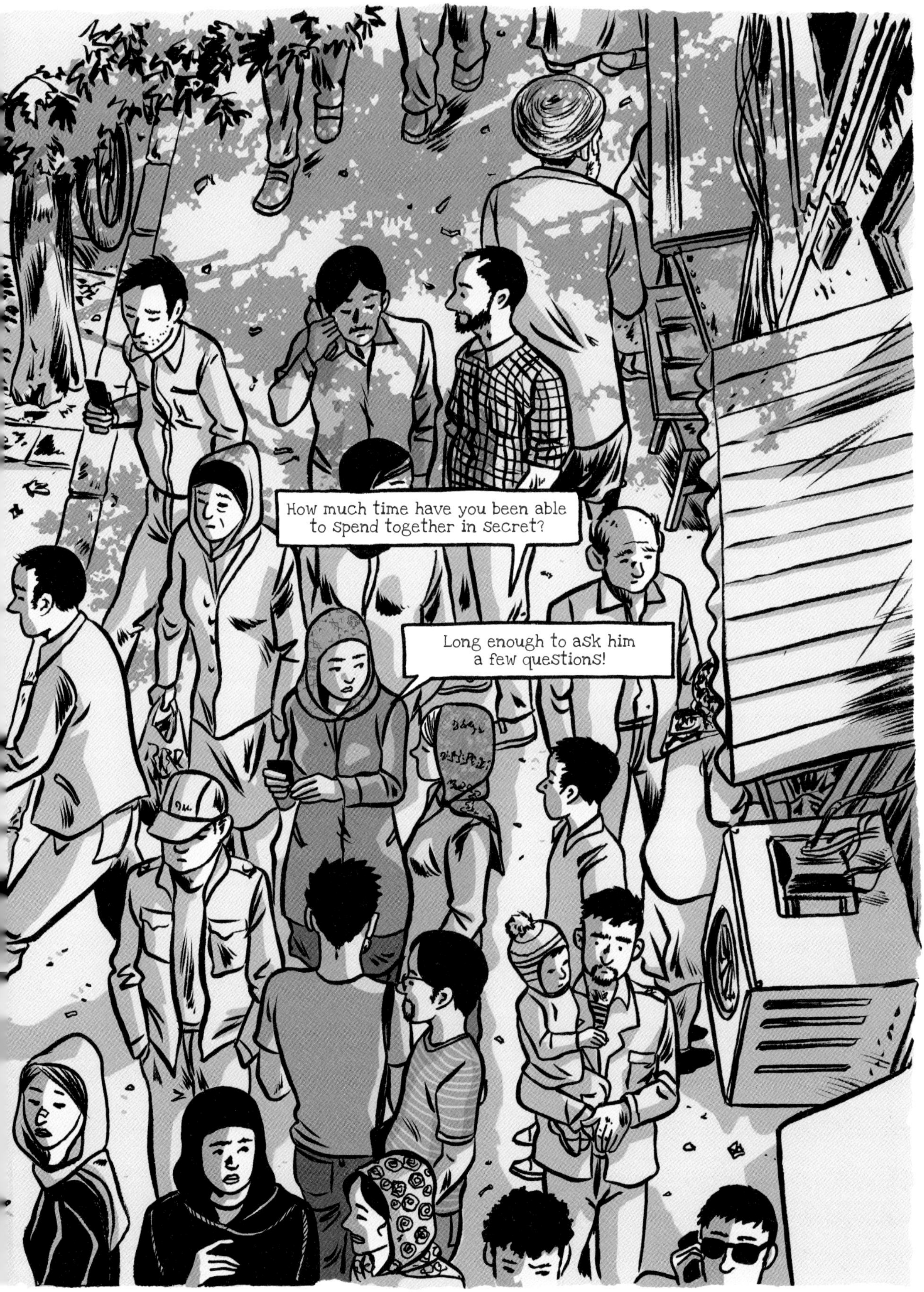
How much time have you been able to spend together in secret?
Long enough to ask him a few questions!

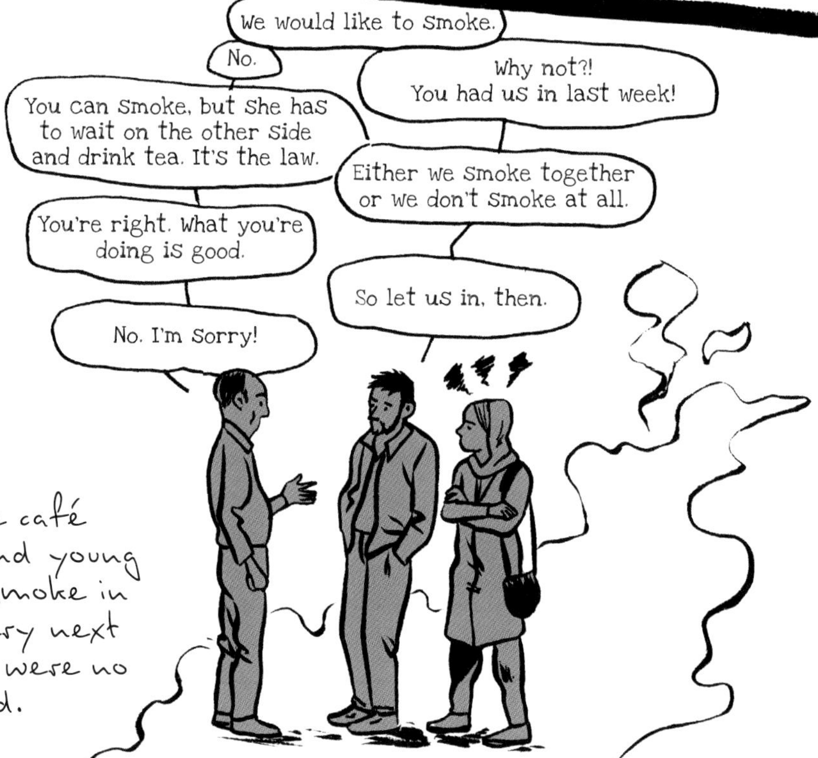
We would like to smoke.
No.
Why not?! You had us in last week!
You can smoke, but she has to wait on the other side and drink tea. It's the law.
Either we smoke together or we don't smoke at all.
You're right. What you're doing is good.
So let us in, then.
No. I'm sorry!

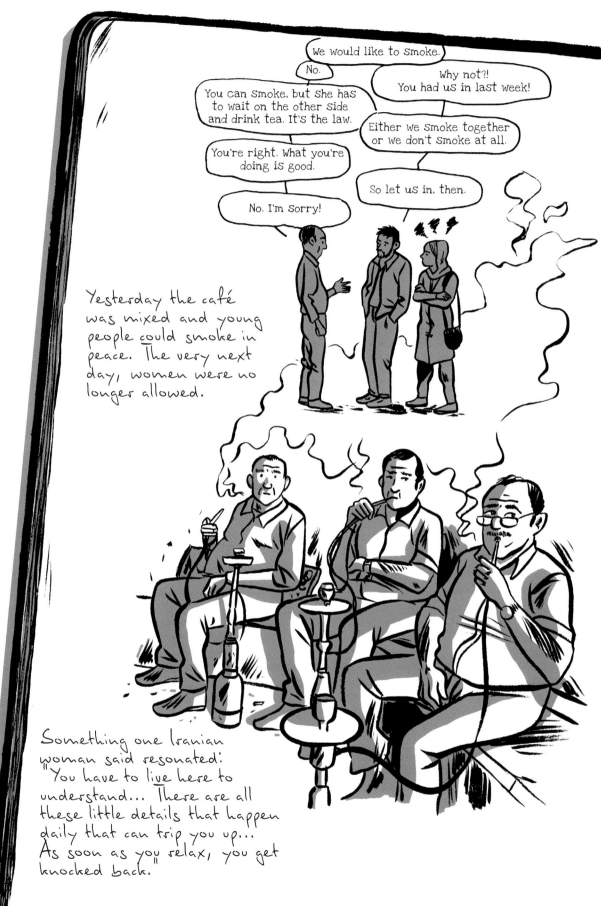

Yesterday the café was mixed and young people could smoke in peace. The very next day, women were no longer allowed.

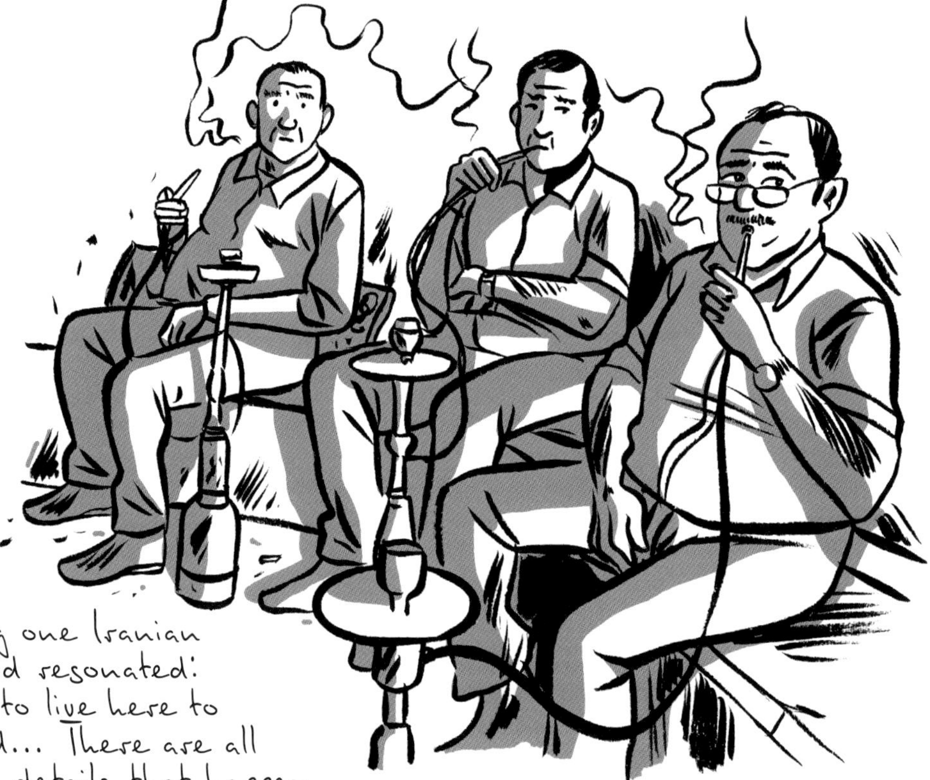

Something one Iranian woman said resonated: "You have to live here to understand... There are all these little details that happen daily that can trip you up... As soon as you relax, you get knocked back."

JAMILEH, 29,
Shiraz.

She has the luxury of breathing the air in Europe.

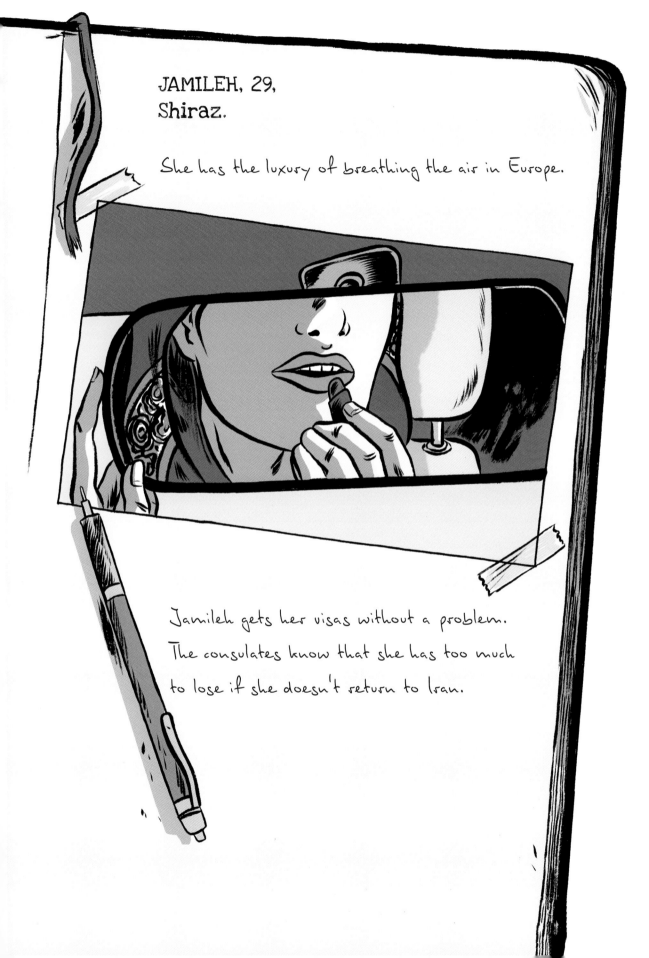

Jamileh gets her visas without a problem.
The consulates know that she has too much
to lose if she doesn't return to Iran.

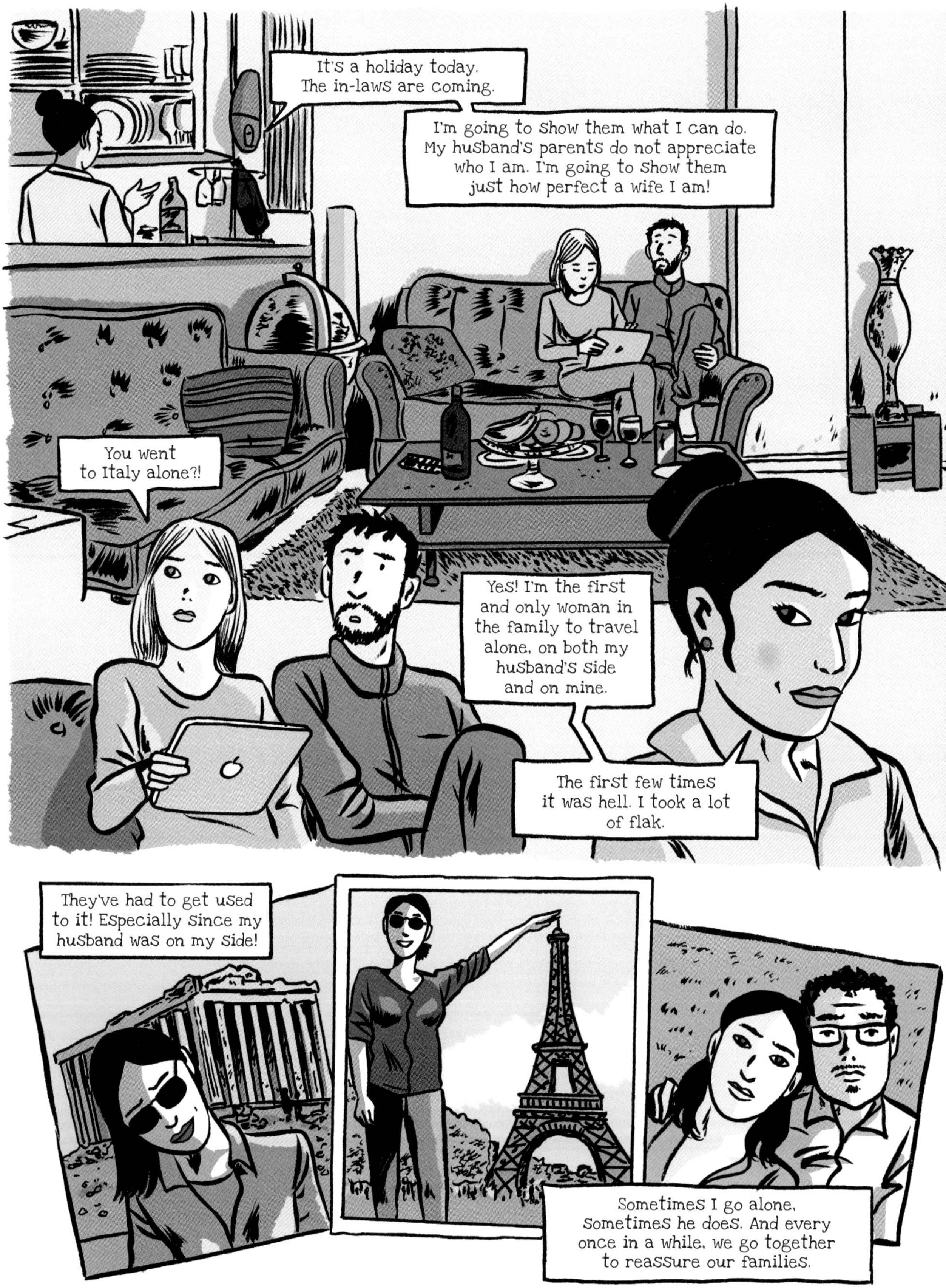
It's a holiday today. The in-laws are coming.
I'm going to show them what I can do. My husband's parents do not appreciate who I am. I'm going to show them just how perfect a wife I am!
You went to Italy alone?!
Yes! I'm the first and only woman in the family to travel alone, on both my husband's side and on mine.
The first few times it was hell. I took a lot of flak.
They've had to get used to it! Especially since my husband was on my side!
Sometimes I go alone, sometimes he does. And every once in a while, we go together to reassure our families.

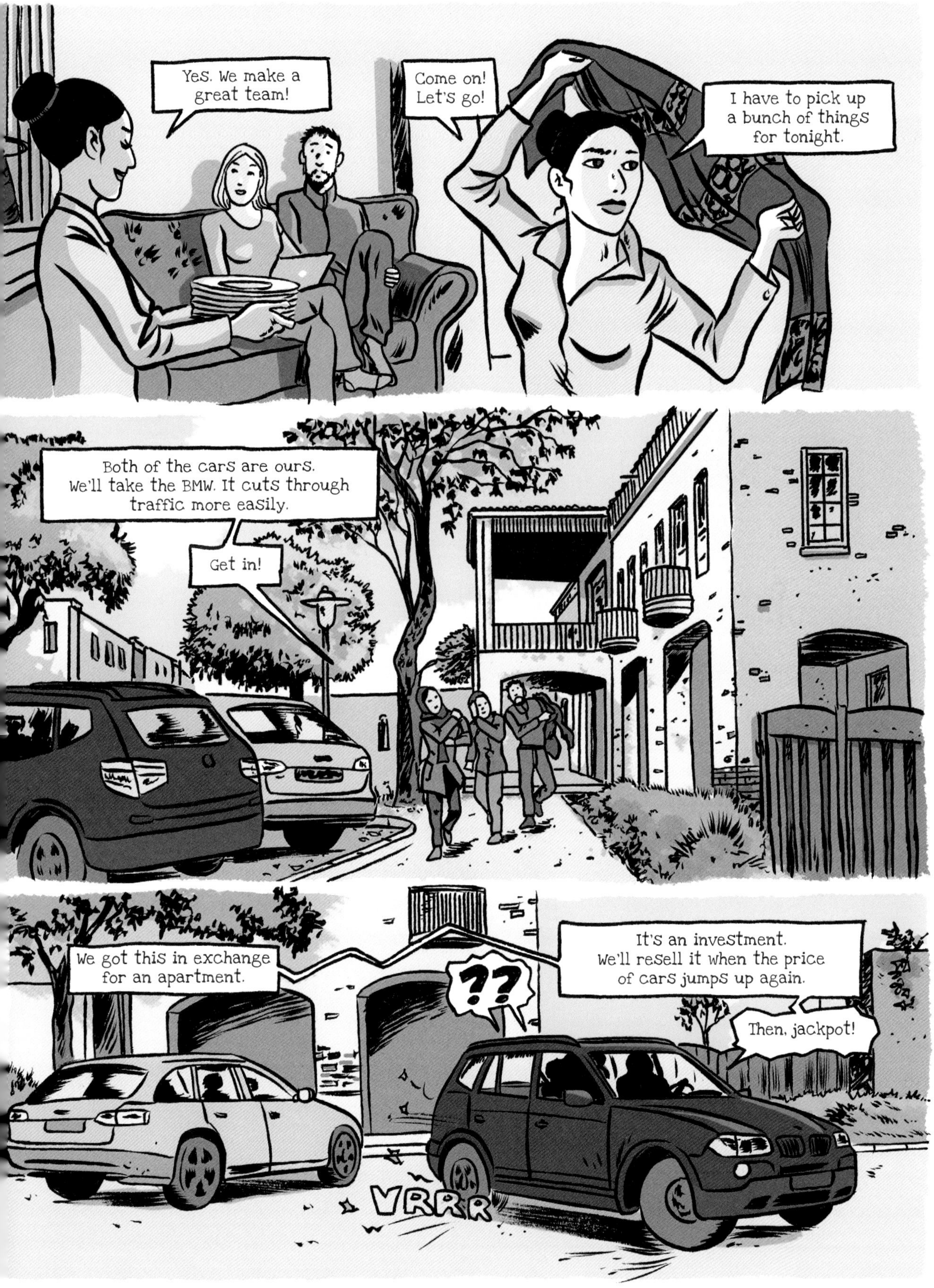
Yes. We make a great team!
Come on! Let's go!
I have to pick up a bunch of things for tonight.
Both of the cars are ours. We'll take the BMW. It cuts through traffic more easily.
Get in!
We got this in exchange for an apartment.
??
It's an investment. We'll resell it when the price of cars jumps up again.
Then, jackpot!
VRRR

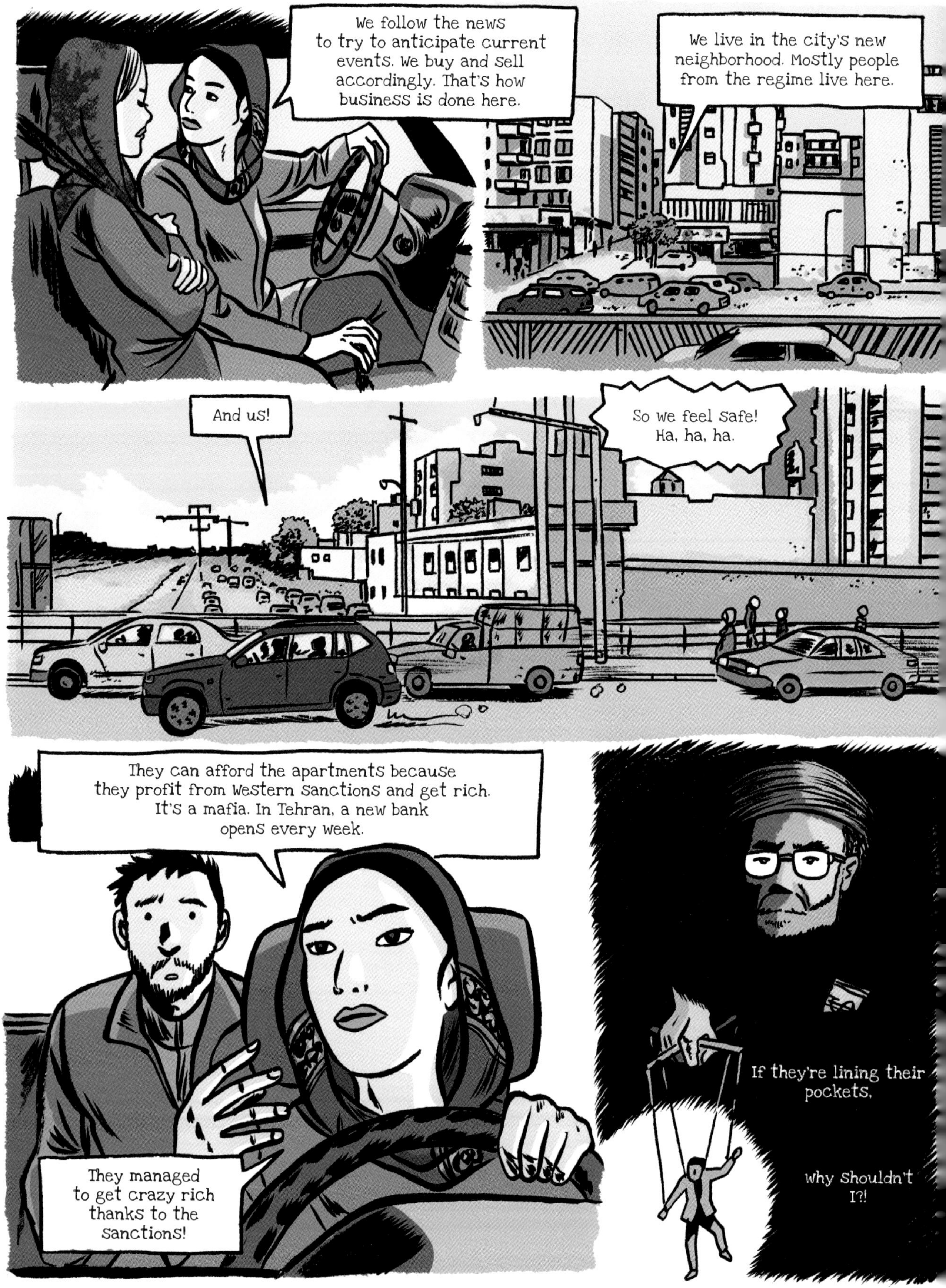
We follow the news to try to anticipate current events. We buy and sell accordingly. That's how business is done here.
We live in the city's new neighborhood. Mostly people from the regime live here.
And us!
So we feel safe! Ha, ha, ha.
They can afford the apartments because they profit from Western sanctions and get rich. It's a mafia. In Tehran, a new bank opens every week.
They managed to get crazy rich thanks to the sanctions!
If they're lining their pockets,
why shouldn't I?!

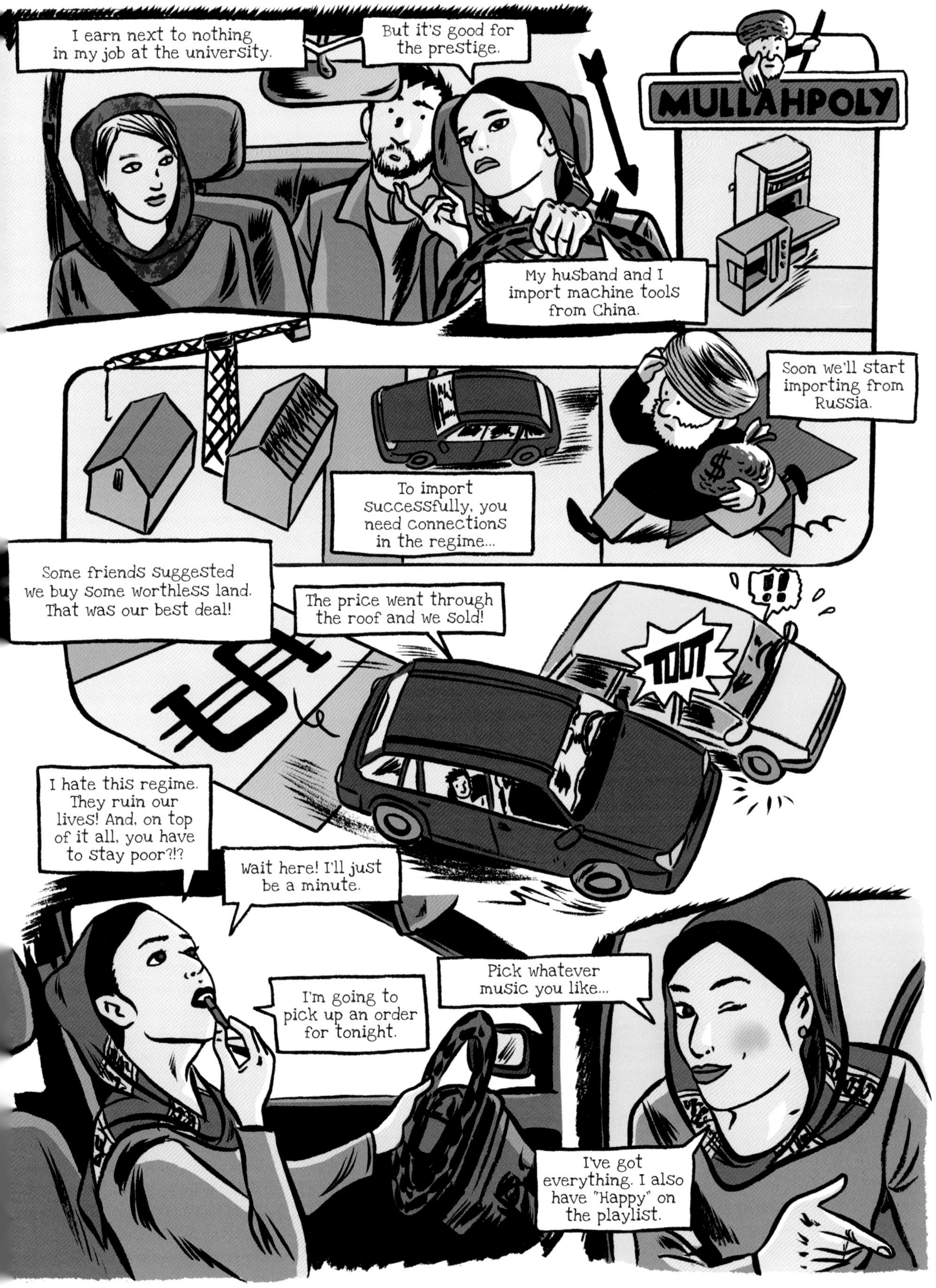
I earn next to nothing in my job at the university.
But it's good for the prestige.
MULLAHPOLY
My husband and I import machine tools from China.
Soon we'll start importing from Russia.
To import successfully, you need connections in the regime...
Some friends suggested we buy some worthless land. That was our best deal!
The price went through the roof and we sold!
!!
TOOT
I hate this regime. They ruin our lives! And, on top of it all, you have to stay poor?!?
Wait here! I'll just be a minute.
I'm going to pick up an order for tonight.
Pick whatever music you like...
I've got everything. I also have "Happy" on the playlist.

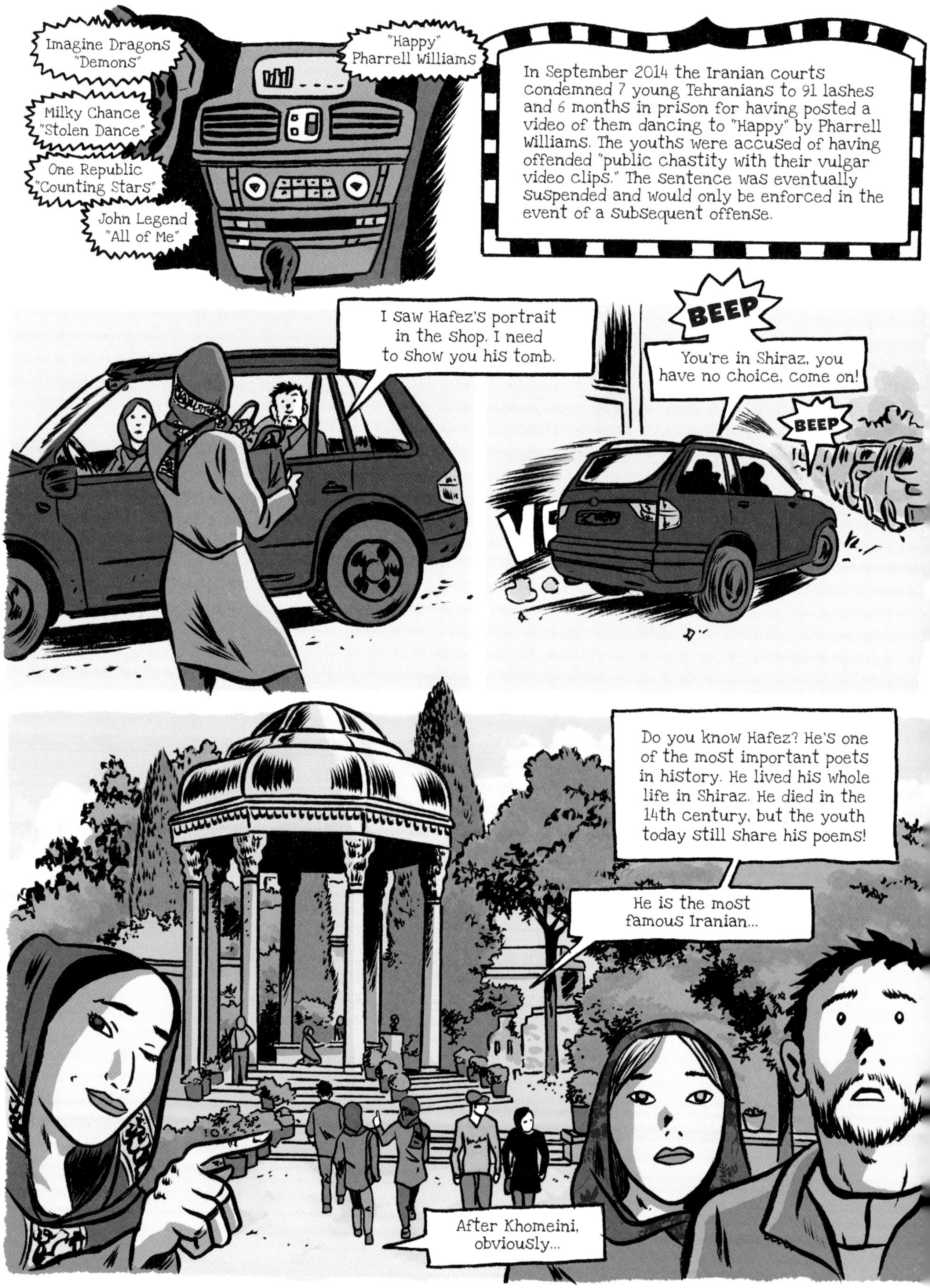
Imagine Dragons "Demons"
Milky Chance "Stolen Dance"
One Republic "Counting Stars"
John Legend "All of Me"
"Happy" Pharrell Williams
In September 2014 the Iranian courts condemned 7 young Tehranians to 91 lashes and 6 months in prison for having posted a video of them dancing to "Happy" by Pharrell Williams. The youths were accused of having offended "public chastity with their vulgar video clips." The sentence was eventually suspended and would only be enforced in the event of a subsequent offense.
I saw Hafez's portrait in the shop. I need to show you his tomb.
BEEP
You're in Shiraz, you have no choice, come on!
BEEP
Do you know Hafez? He's one of the most important poets in history. He lived his whole life in Shiraz. He died in the 14th century, but the youth today still share his poems!
He is the most famous Iranian...
After Khomeini, obviously...

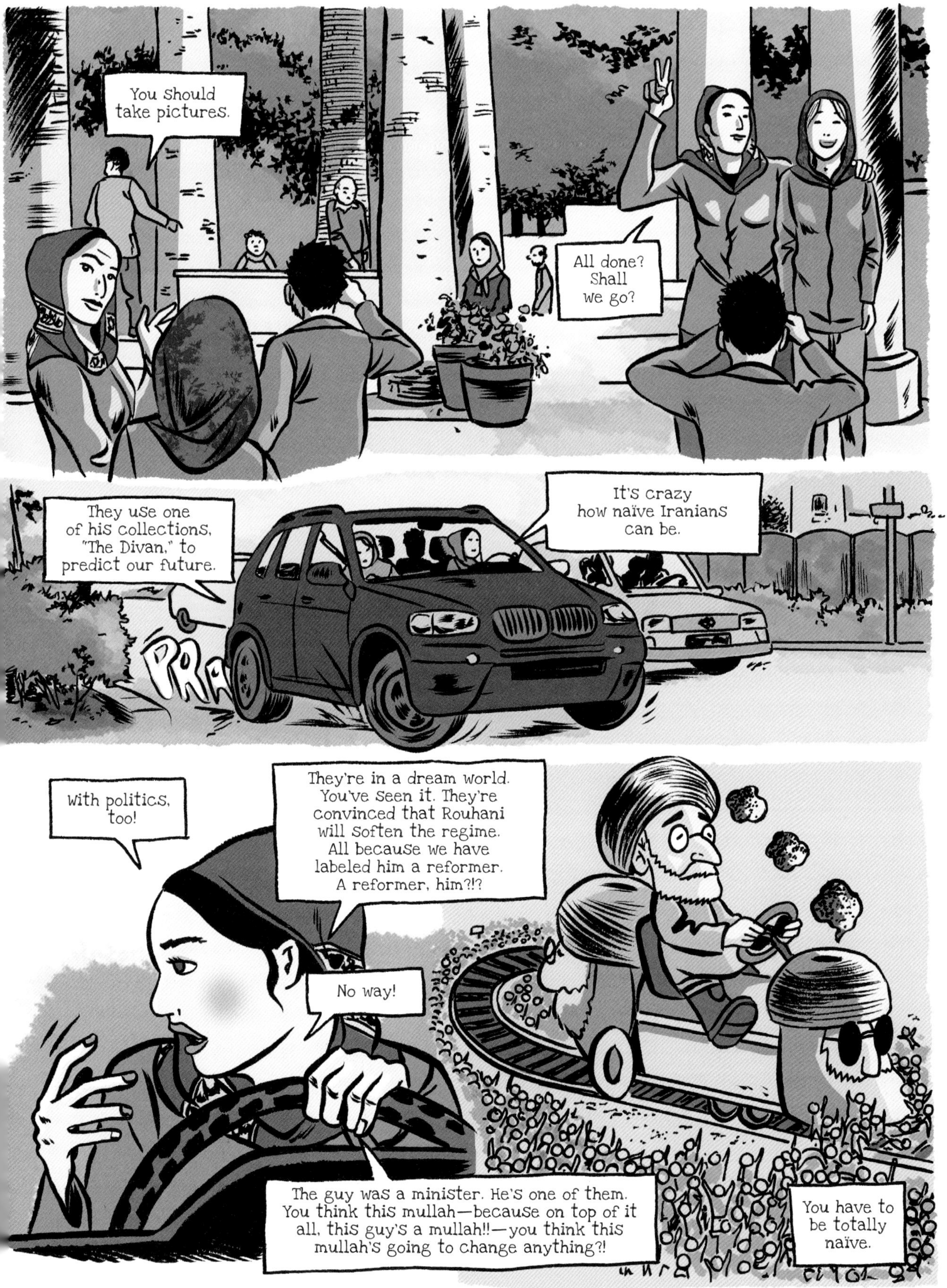
You should take pictures.
All done? Shall we go?
They use one of his collections, "The Divan," to predict our future.
It's crazy how naïve Iranians can be.
PRA
With politics, too!
They're in a dream world. You've seen it. They're convinced that Rouhani will soften the regime. All because we have labeled him a reformer. A reformer, him?!?
No way!
The guy was a minister. He's one of them. You think this mullah—because on top of it all, this guy's a mullah!!—you think this mullah's going to change anything?!
You have to be totally naïve.

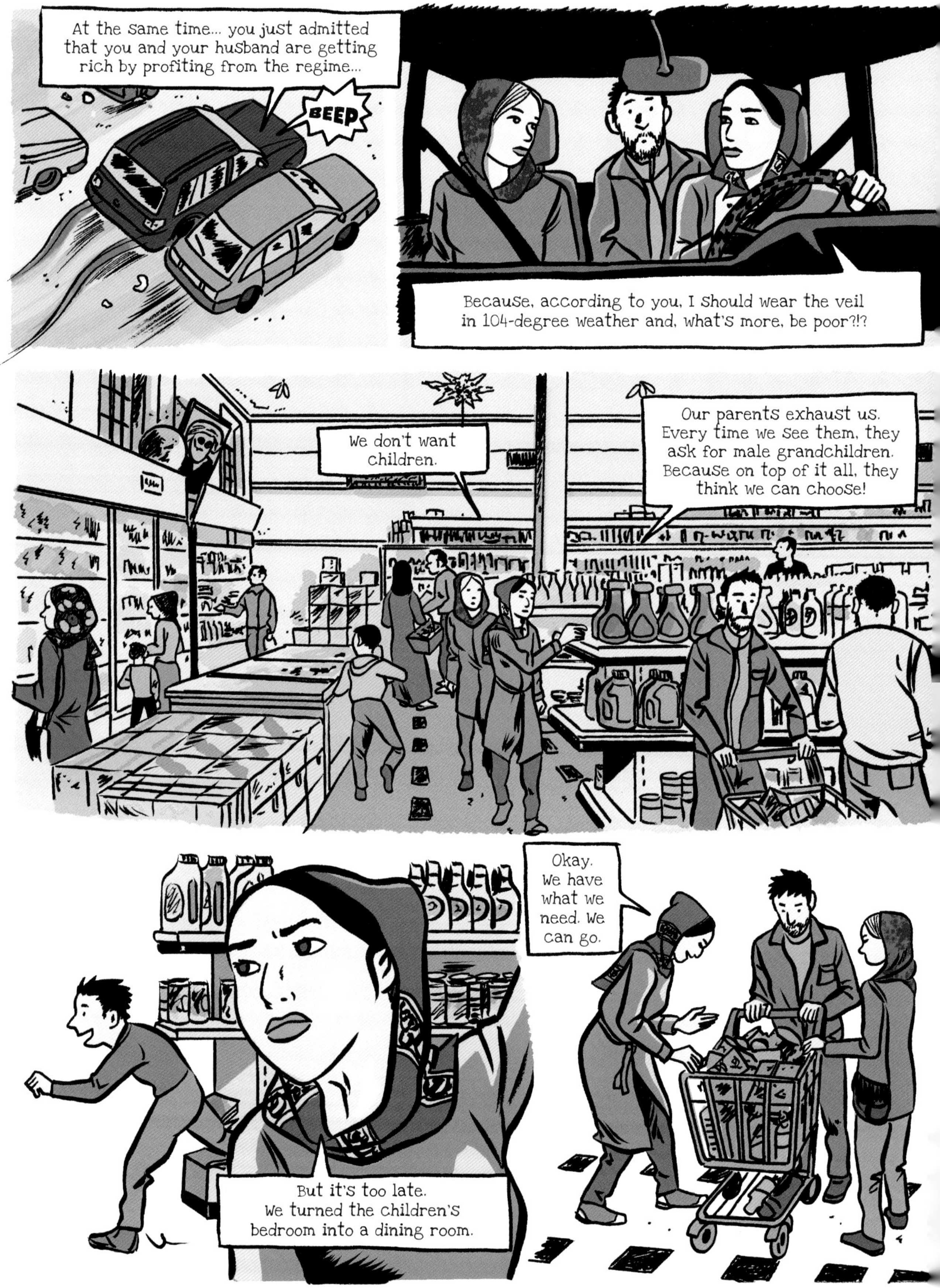
At the same time... you just admitted that you and your husband are getting rich by profiting from the regime...
BEEP
Because, according to you, I should wear the veil in 104-degree weather and, what's more, be poor?!?
We don't want children.
Our parents exhaust us. Every time we see them, they ask for male grandchildren. Because on top of it all, they think we can choose!
But it's too late. We turned the children's bedroom into a dining room.
Okay. We have what we need. We can go.

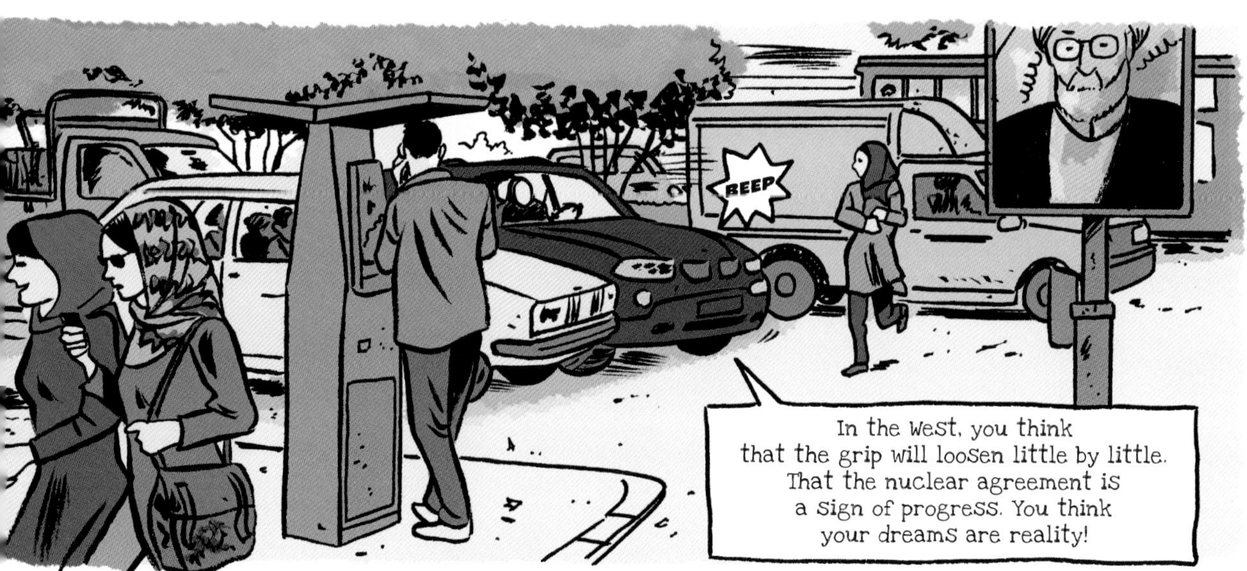
BEEP
In the West, you think that the grip will loosen little by little. That the nuclear agreement is a sign of progress. You think your dreams are reality!

It's really just the opposite.

Rouhani wants to put Iran back on the international scene and relaunch the economy. If Iranians can eat and buy what they want, they won't demonstrate. We will perhaps be richer, but not freer. Besides, there are laws being drafted to make our lives even more difficult than they are now.

These people know how to organize things.

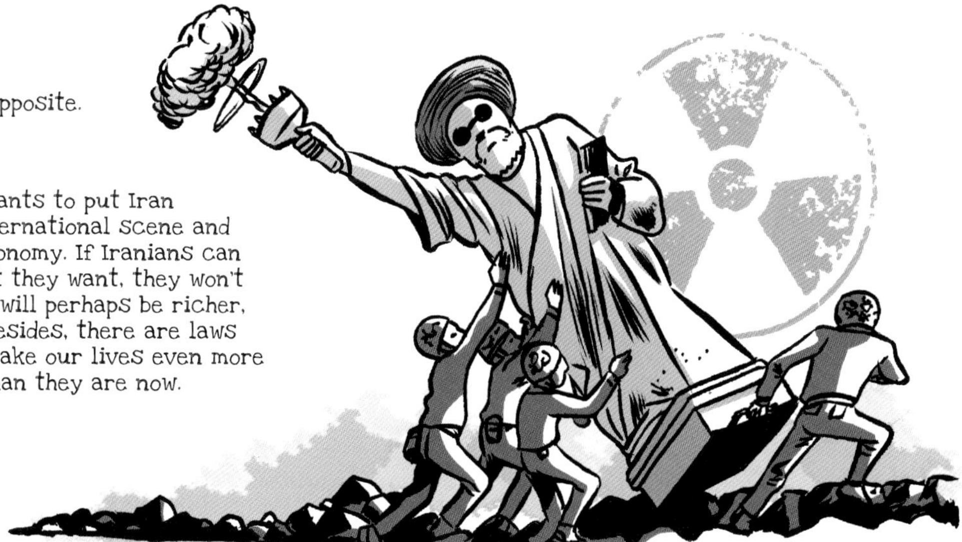

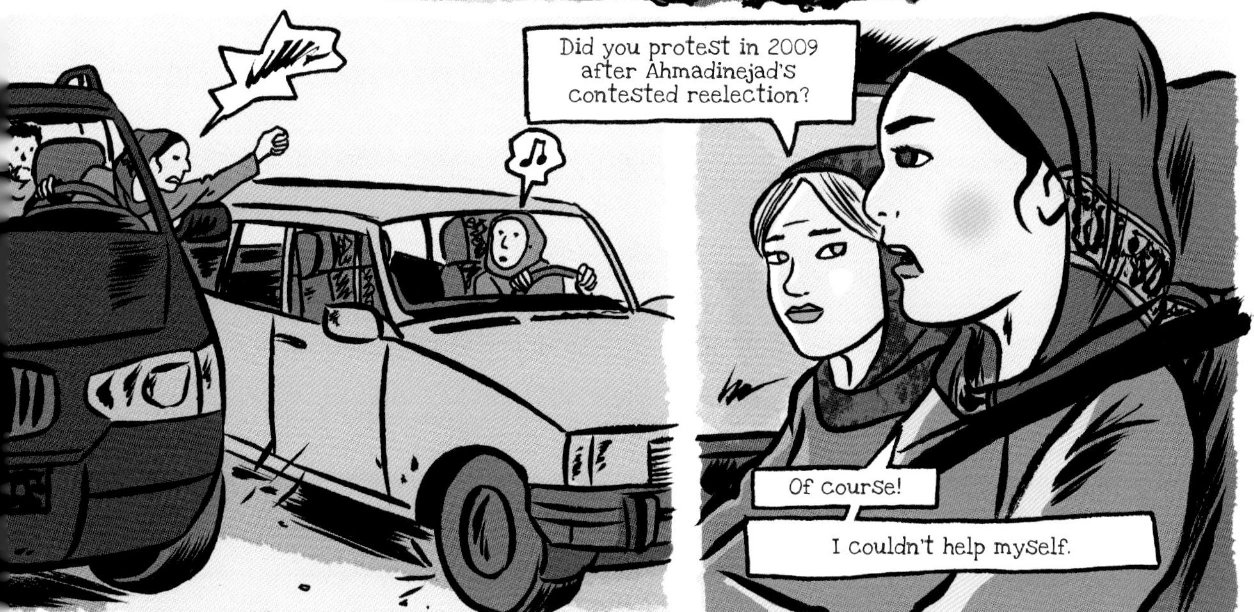
Did you protest in 2009 after Ahmadinejad's contested reelection?
Of course!
I couldn't help myself.

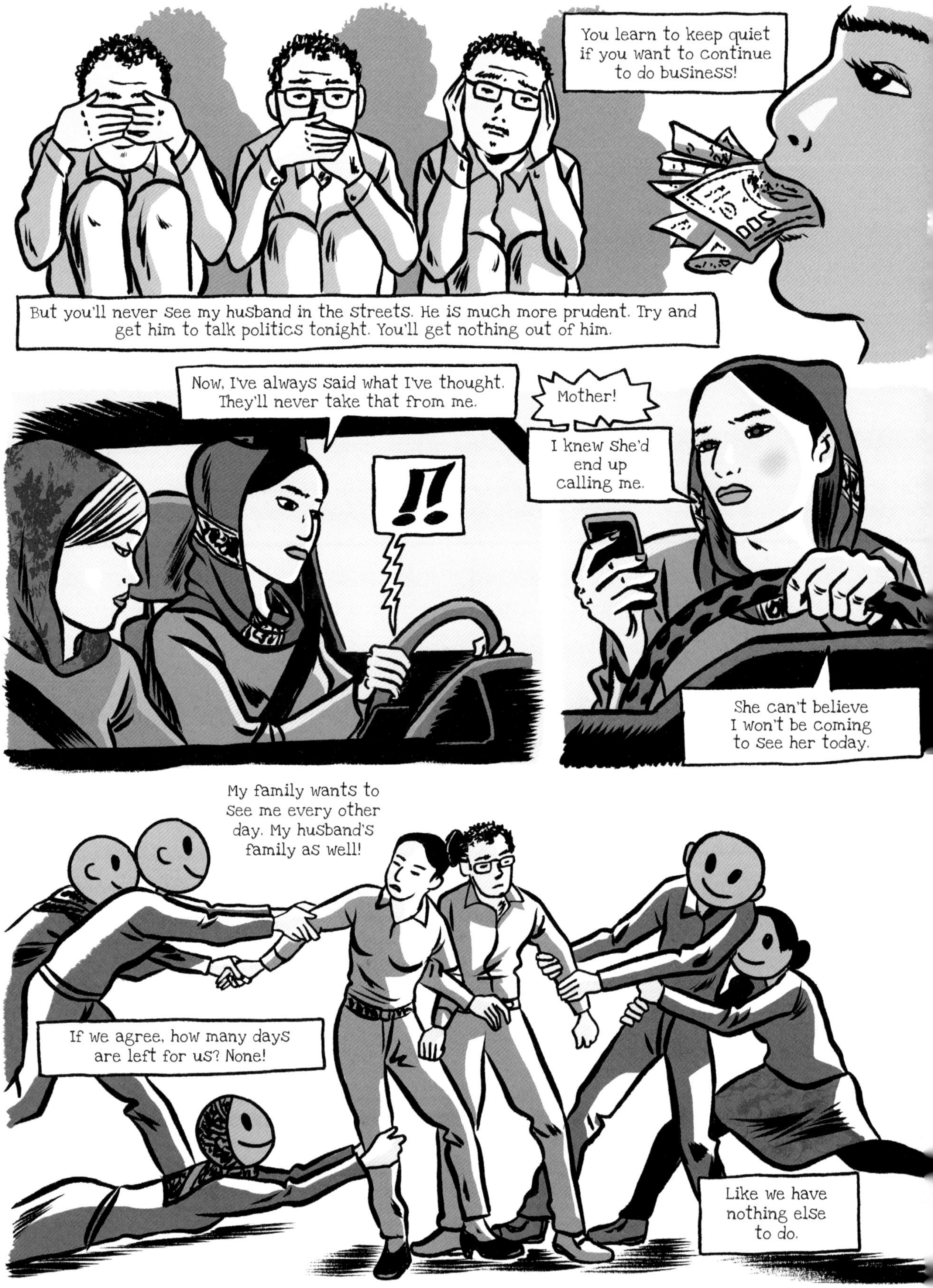
You learn to keep quiet if you want to continue to do business!
But you'll never see my husband in the streets. He is much more prudent. Try and get him to talk politics tonight. You'll get nothing out of him.
Now, I've always said what I've thought. They'll never take that from me.
!!
Mother!
I knew she'd end up calling me.
She can't believe I won't be coming to see her today.
My family wants to see me every other day. My husband's family as well!
If we agree, how many days are left for us? None!
Like we have nothing else to do.

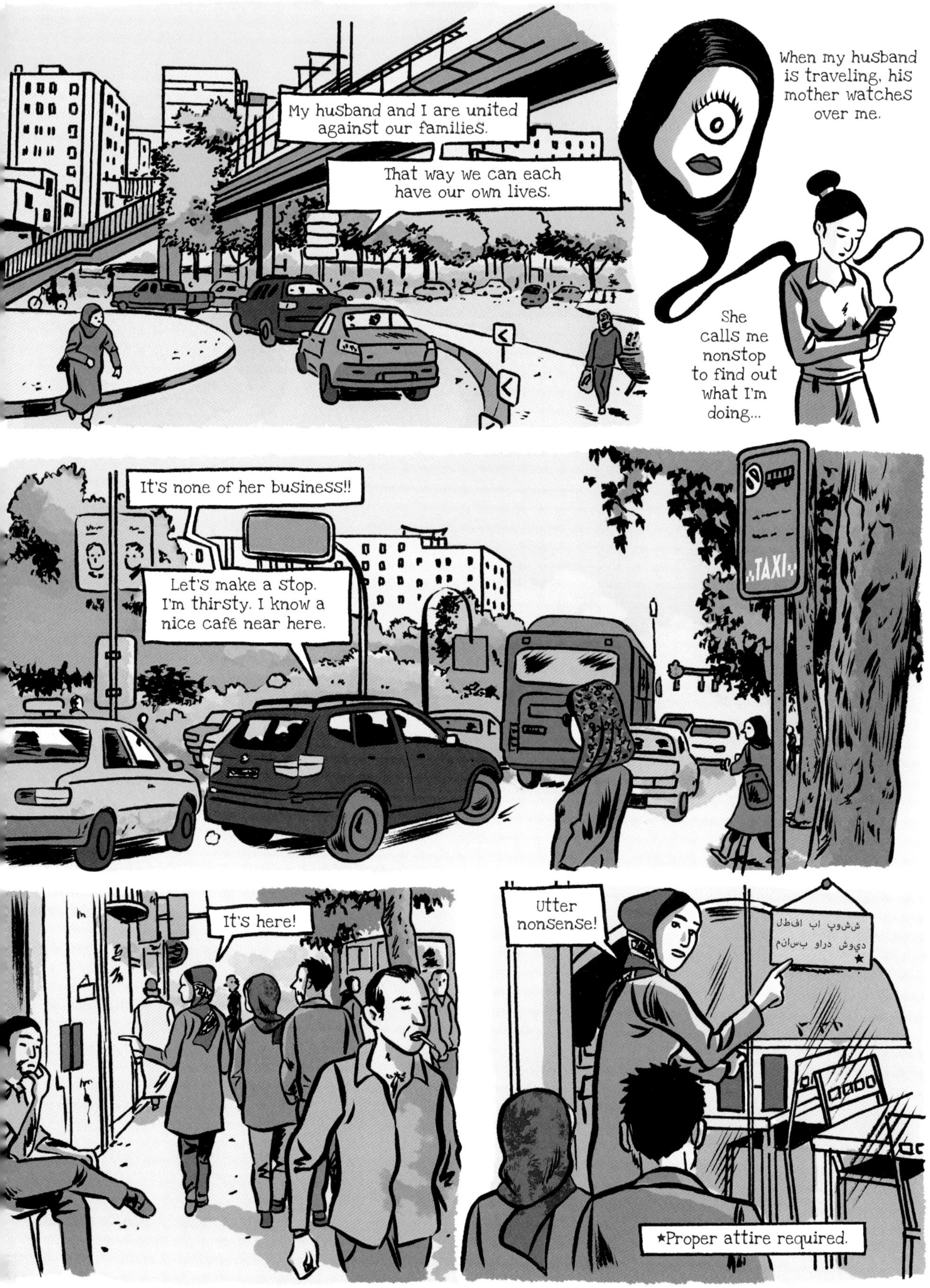

My husband and I are united against our families.
That way we can each have our own lives.
When my husband is traveling, his mother watches over me.
She calls me nonstop to find out what I'm doing...
It's none of her business!!
Let's make a stop. I'm thirsty. I know a nice café near here.
TAXI
It's here!
Utter nonsense!
★Proper attire required.

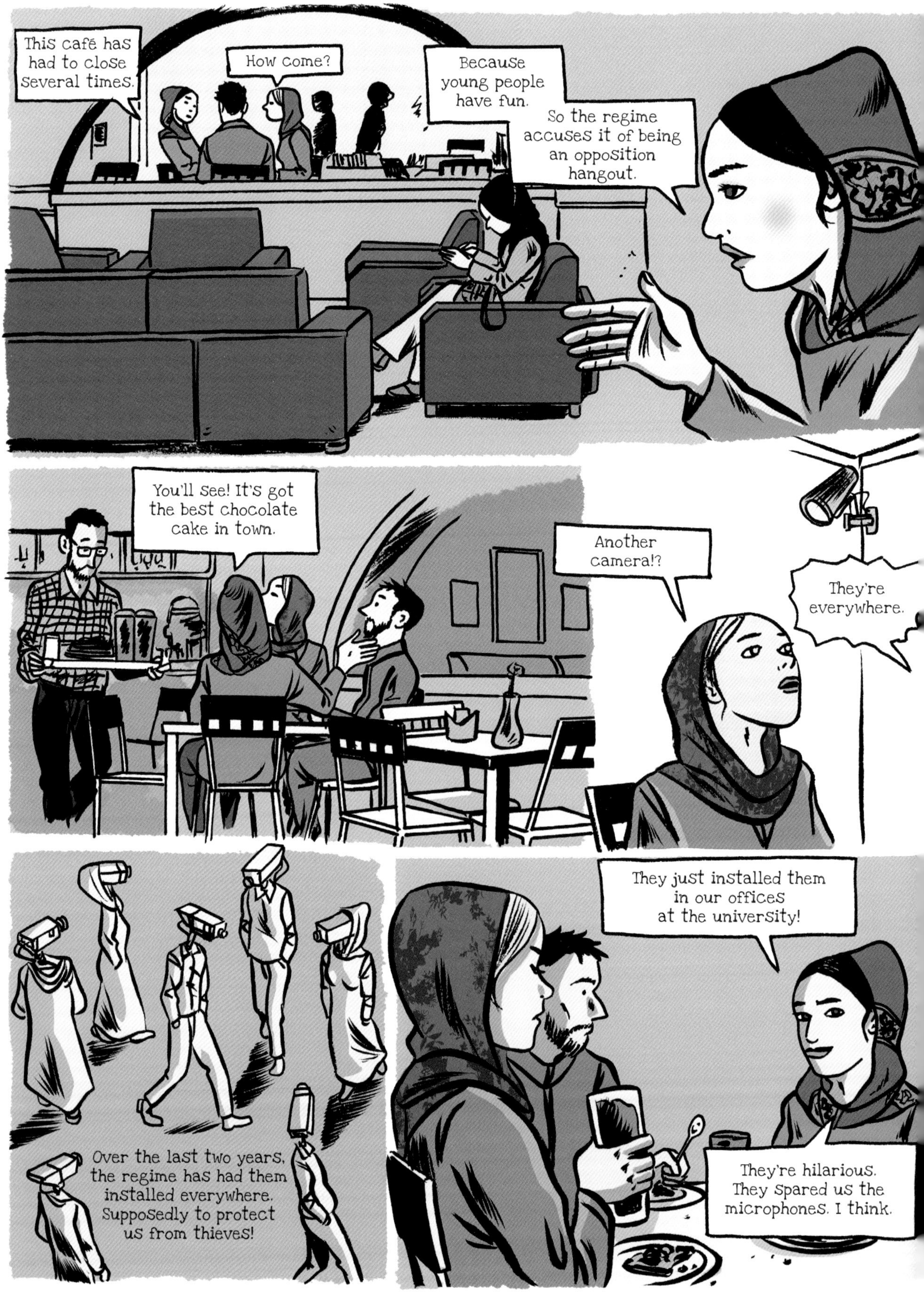
This café has had to close several times.
How come?
Because young people have fun.
So the regime accuses it of being an opposition hangout.
You'll see! It's got the best chocolate cake in town.
Another camera!?
They're everywhere.
Over the last two years, the regime has had them installed everywhere. Supposedly to protect us from thieves!
They just installed them in our offices at the university!
They're hilarious. They spared us the microphones. I think.

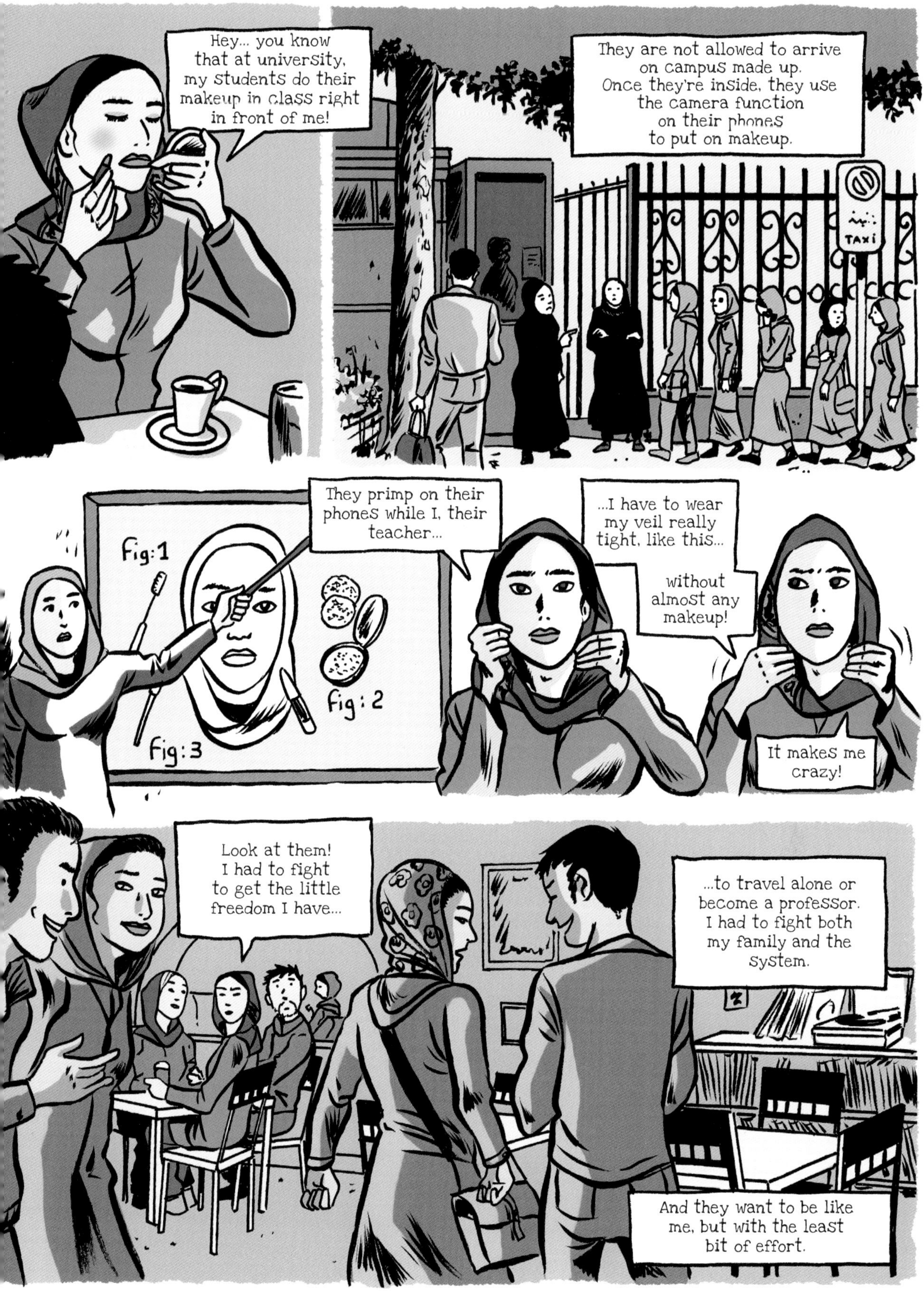
Hey... you know that at university, my students do their makeup in class right in front of me!
They are not allowed to arrive on campus made up. Once they're inside, they use the camera function on their phones to put on makeup.
TAXI
They primp on their phones while I, their teacher...
Fig: 1
Fig: 2
Fig: 3
...I have to wear my veil really tight, like this...
without almost any makeup!
It makes me crazy!
Look at them! I had to fight to get the little freedom I have...
...to travel alone or become a professor. I had to fight both my family and the system.
And they want to be like me, but with the least bit of effort.

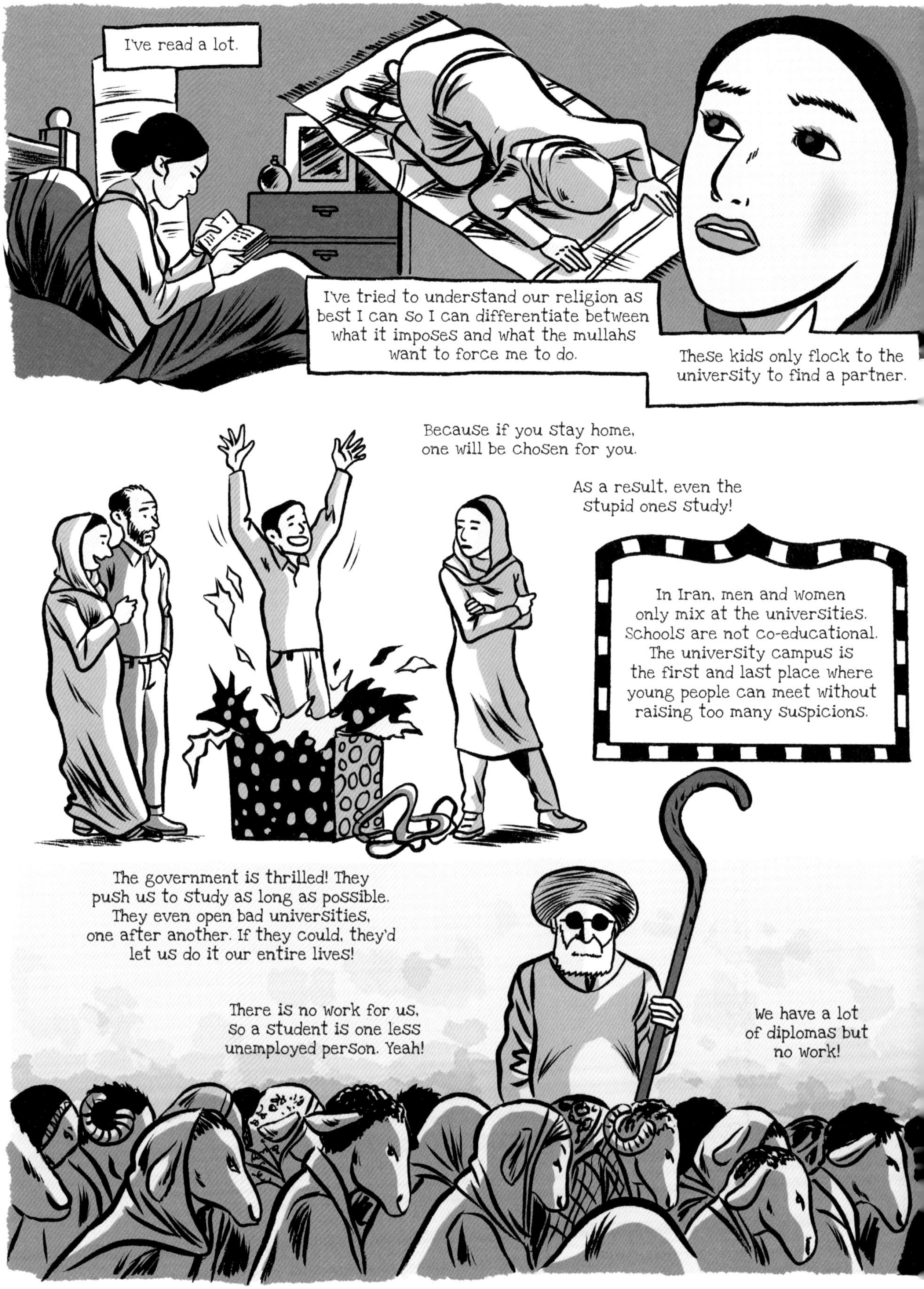
I've read a lot.
I've tried to understand our religion as best I can so I can differentiate between what it imposes and what the mullahs want to force me to do.
These kids only flock to the university to find a partner.
Because if you stay home, one will be chosen for you.
As a result, even the stupid ones study!
In Iran, men and women only mix at the universities. Schools are not co-educational. The university campus is the first and last place where young people can meet without raising too many suspicions.
The government is thrilled! They push us to study as long as possible. They even open bad universities, one after another. If they could, they'd let us do it our entire lives!
There is no work for us, so a student is one less unemployed person. Yeah!
We have a lot of diplomas but no work!

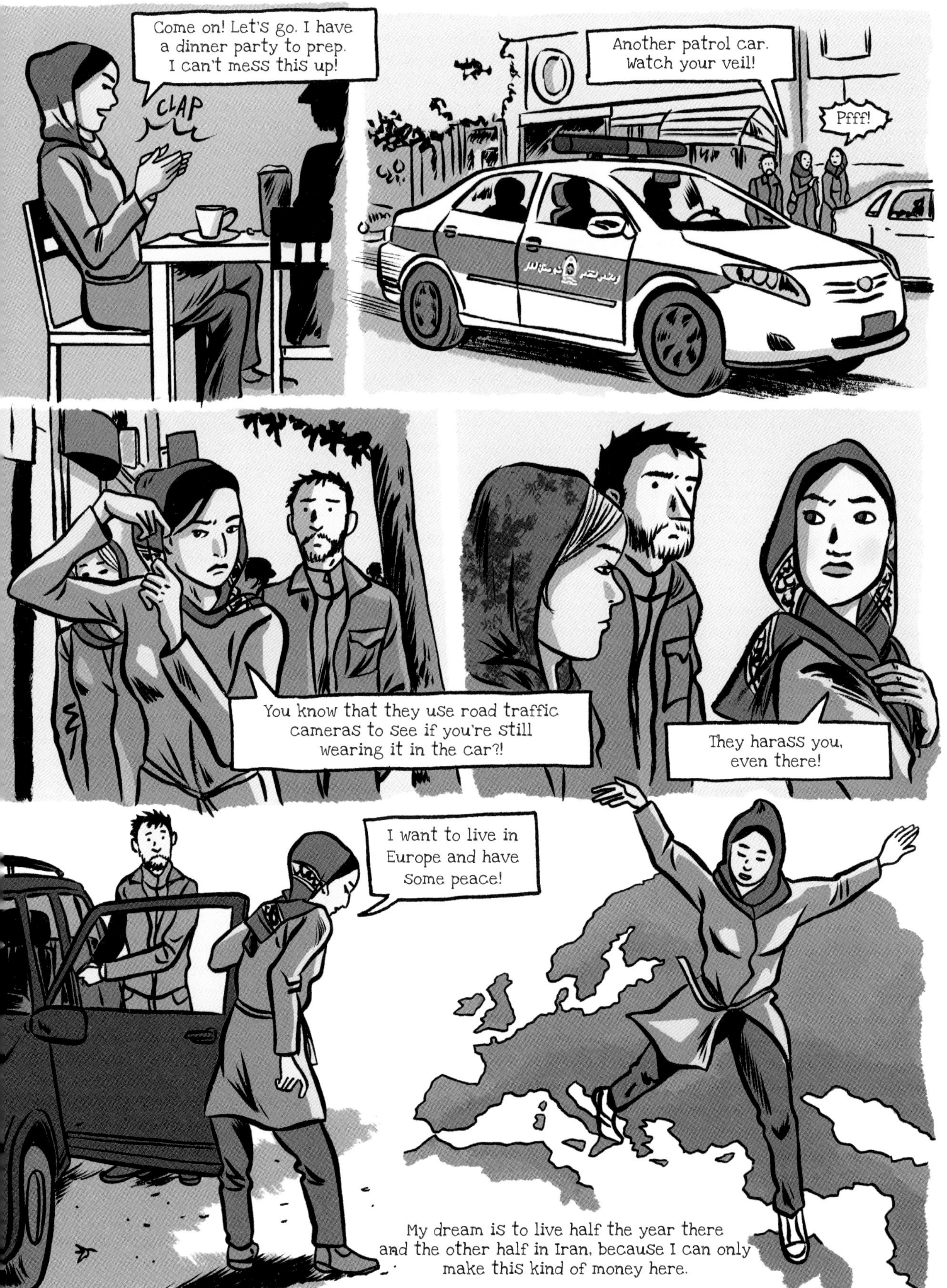
Come on! Let's go. I have a dinner party to prep. I can't mess this up!
CLAP
Another patrol car. Watch your veil!
Pfff!
You know that they use road traffic cameras to see if you're still wearing it in the car?!
They harass you, even there!
I want to live in Europe and have some peace!
My dream is to live half the year there and the other half in Iran, because I can only make this kind of money here.

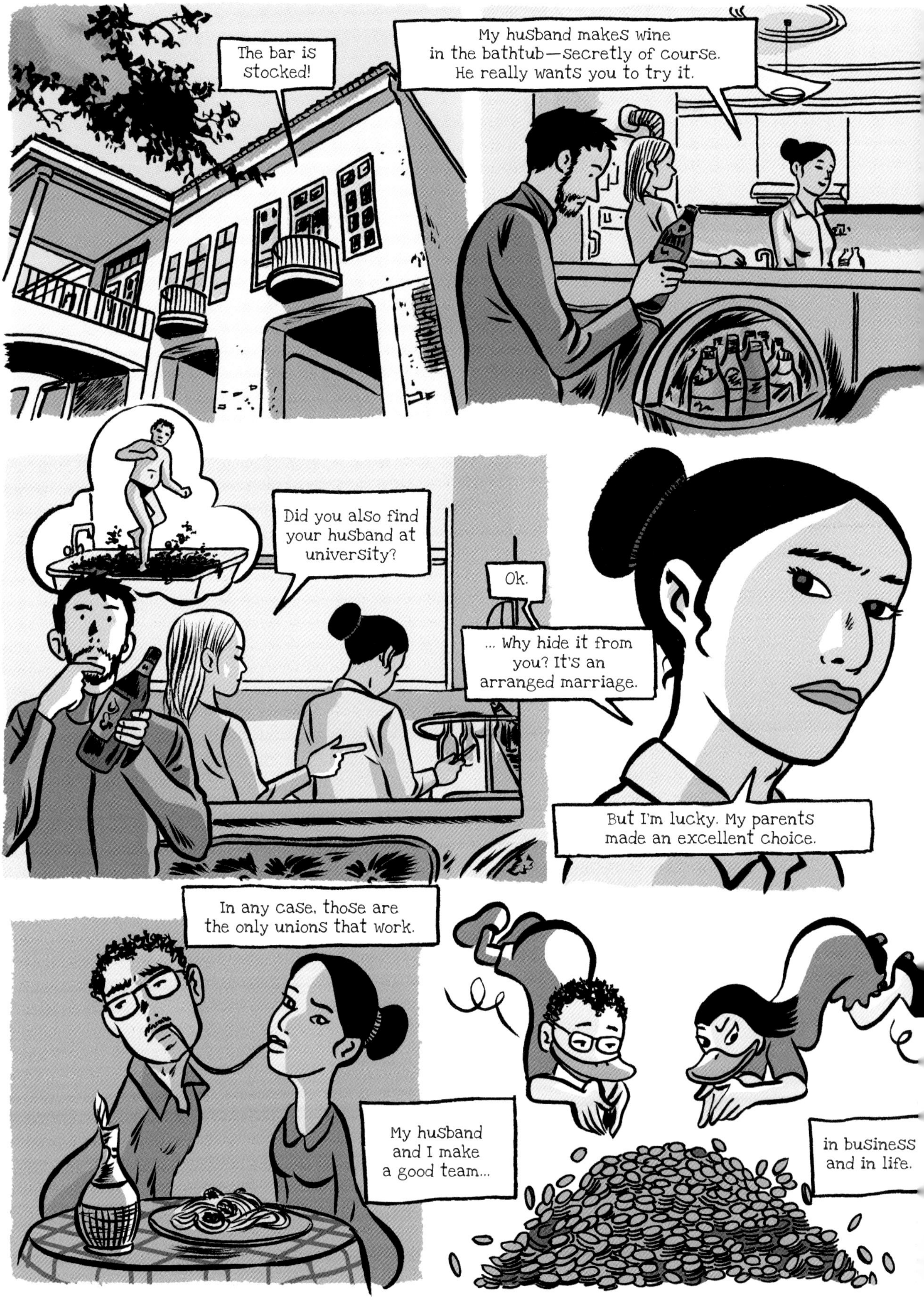
The bar is stocked!
My husband makes wine in the bathtub—secretly of course. He really wants you to try it.
Did you also find your husband at university?
Ok.
... Why hide it from you? It's an arranged marriage.
But I'm lucky. My parents made an excellent choice.
In any case, those are the only unions that work.
My husband and I make a good team...
in business and in life.

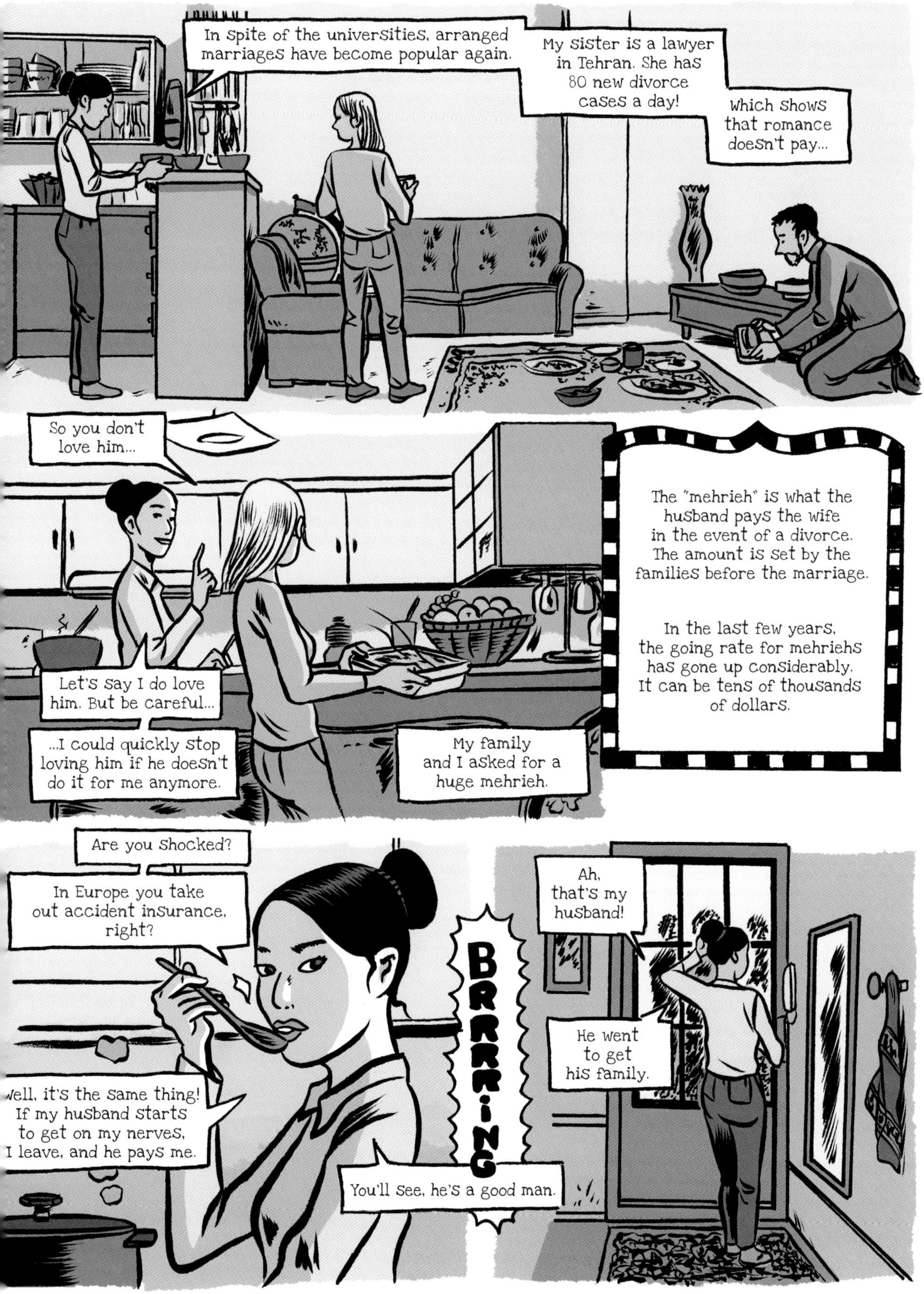

In spite of the universities, arranged marriages have become popular again.
My sister is a lawyer in Tehran. She has 80 new divorce cases a day!
Which shows that romance doesn't pay...
So you don't love him...
The "mehrieh" is what the husband pays the wife in the event of a divorce. The amount is set by the families before the marriage.
In the last few years, the going rate for mehriehs has gone up considerably. It can be tens of thousands of dollars.
Let's say I do love him. But be careful...
...I could quickly stop loving him if he doesn't do it for me anymore.
My family and I asked for a huge mehrieh.
Are you shocked?
In Europe you take out accident insurance, right?
Well, it's the same thing! If my husband starts to get on my nerves, I leave, and he pays me.
BRRRRiNG
You'll see, he's a good man.
Ah, that's my husband!
He went to get his family.

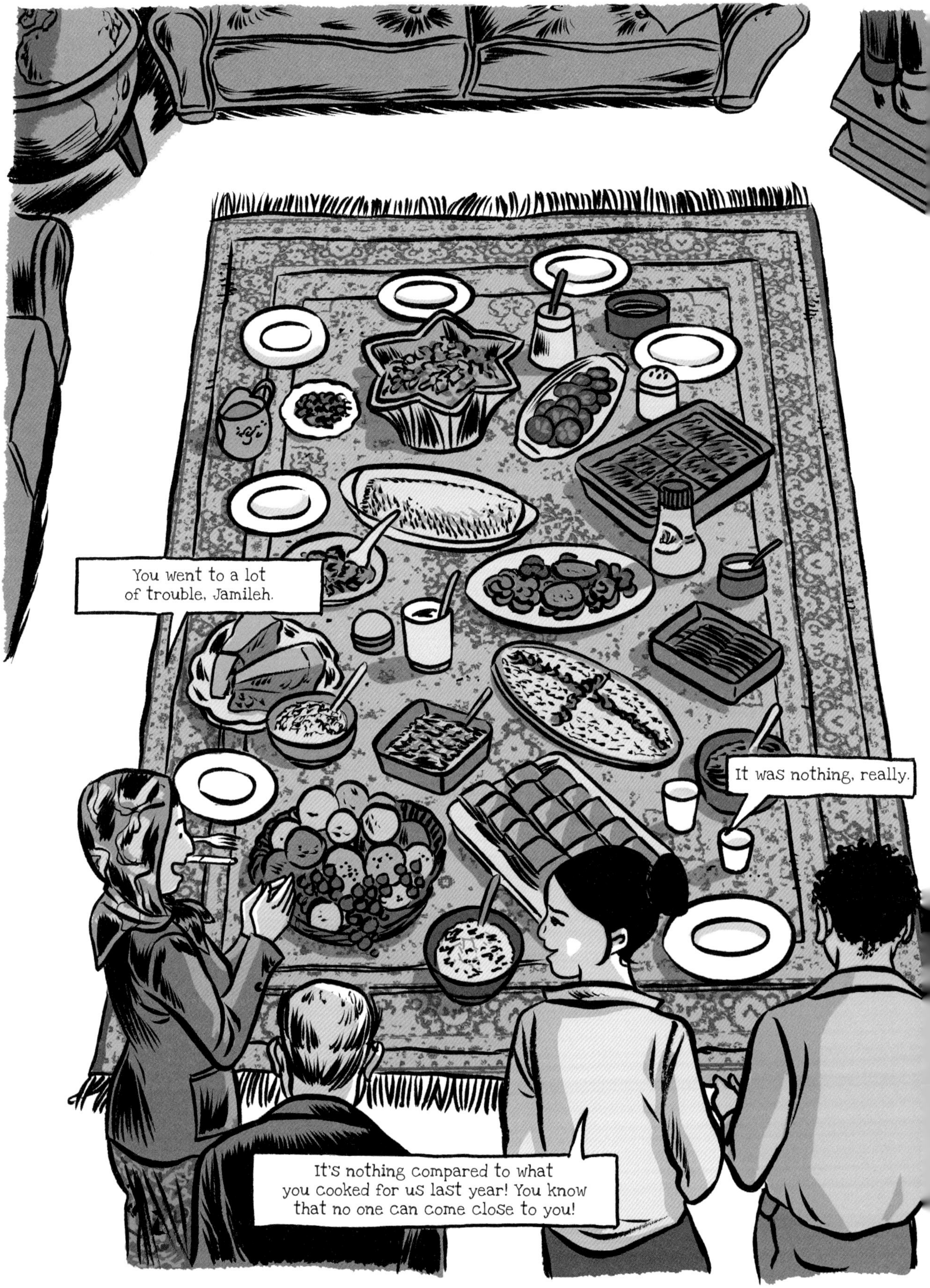
You went to a lot of trouble, Jamileh.
It was nothing, really.
It's nothing compared to what you cooked for us last year! You know that no one can come close to you!

A few days later, in the Tehran Museum of Contemporary Art, one or two Iranians wander around alone.

You'll let me know if you want to move in with me.
But at the same time, it's nice for each of us to have our own space...
...

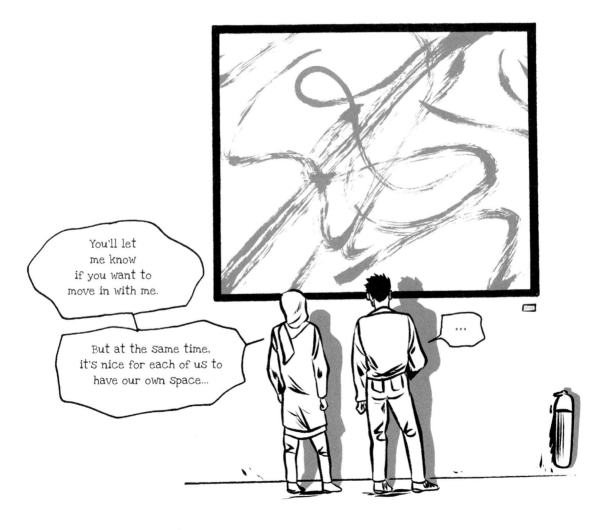

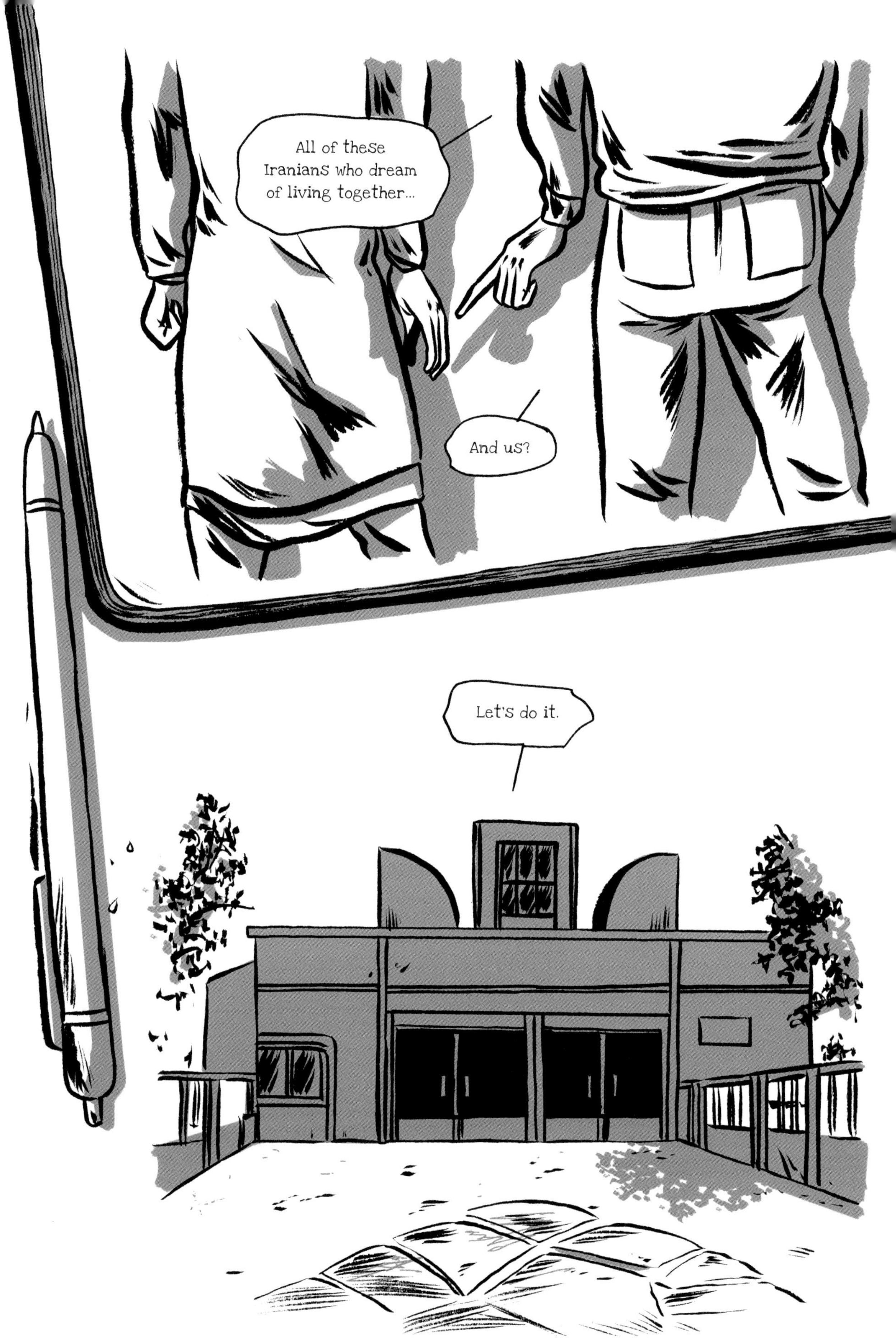
All of these Iranians who dream of living together...
And us?
Let's do it.

LEILA, 26,
Tehran.

A few hours before our
departure, we met with
people from Iranian
high society. These people
were 20 in 1979.

For them, much has changed
since then. But they see little
evolution in Iran in general
over the last 35 years.
Life is still deeply rooted
in tradition.

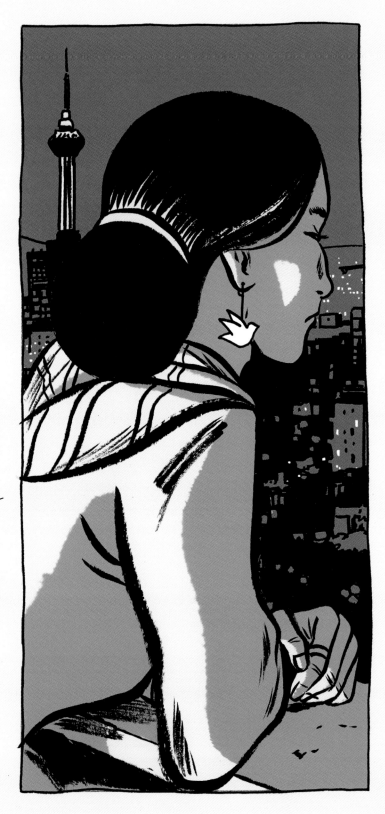

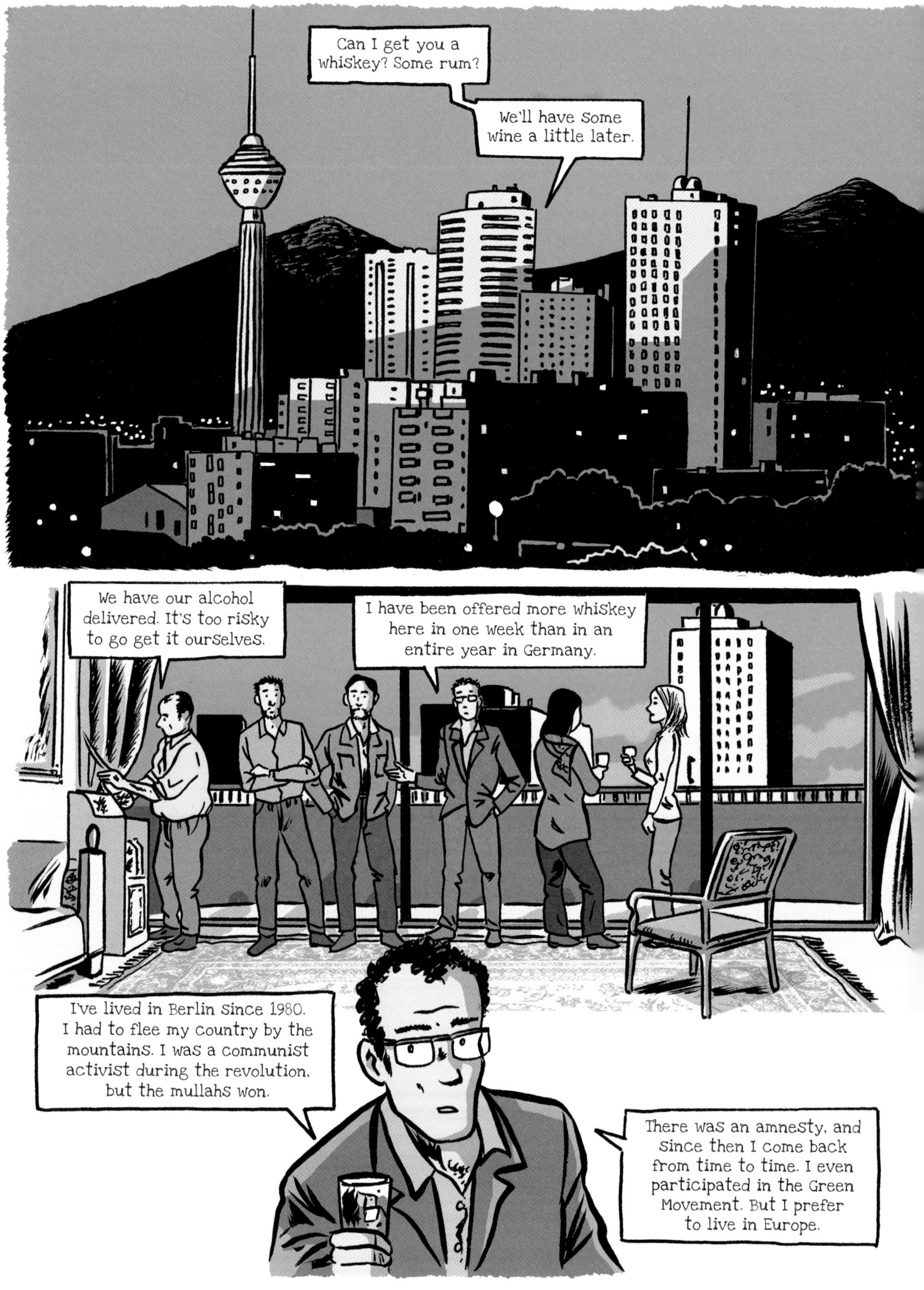
Can I get you a whiskey? Some rum?
We'll have some wine a little later.
We have our alcohol delivered. It's too risky to go get it ourselves.
I have been offered more whiskey here in one week than in an entire year in Germany.
I've lived in Berlin since 1980. I had to flee my country by the mountains. I was a communist activist during the revolution, but the mullahs won.
There was an amnesty, and since then I come back from time to time. I even participated in the Green Movement. But I prefer to live in Europe.

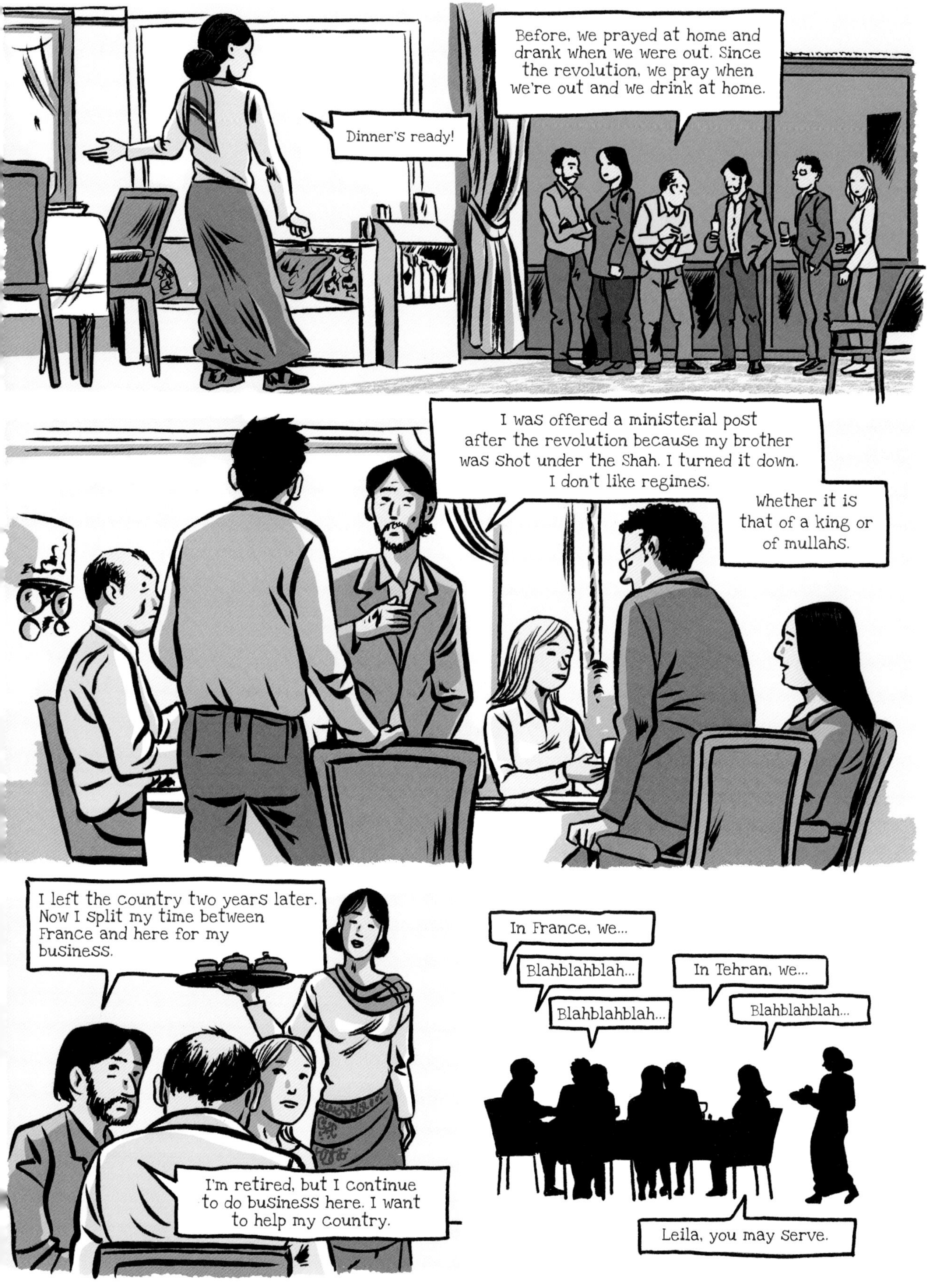
Before, we prayed at home and drank when we were out. Since the revolution, we pray when we're out and we drink at home.
Dinner's ready!
I was offered a ministerial post after the revolution because my brother was shot under the Shah. I turned it down. I don't like regimes.
Whether it is that of a king or of mullahs.
I left the country two years later. Now I split my time between France and here for my business.
I'm retired, but I continue to do business here. I want to help my country.
In France, we...
Blahblahblah...
Blahblahblah...
In Tehran, we...
Blahblahblah...
Leila, you may serve.

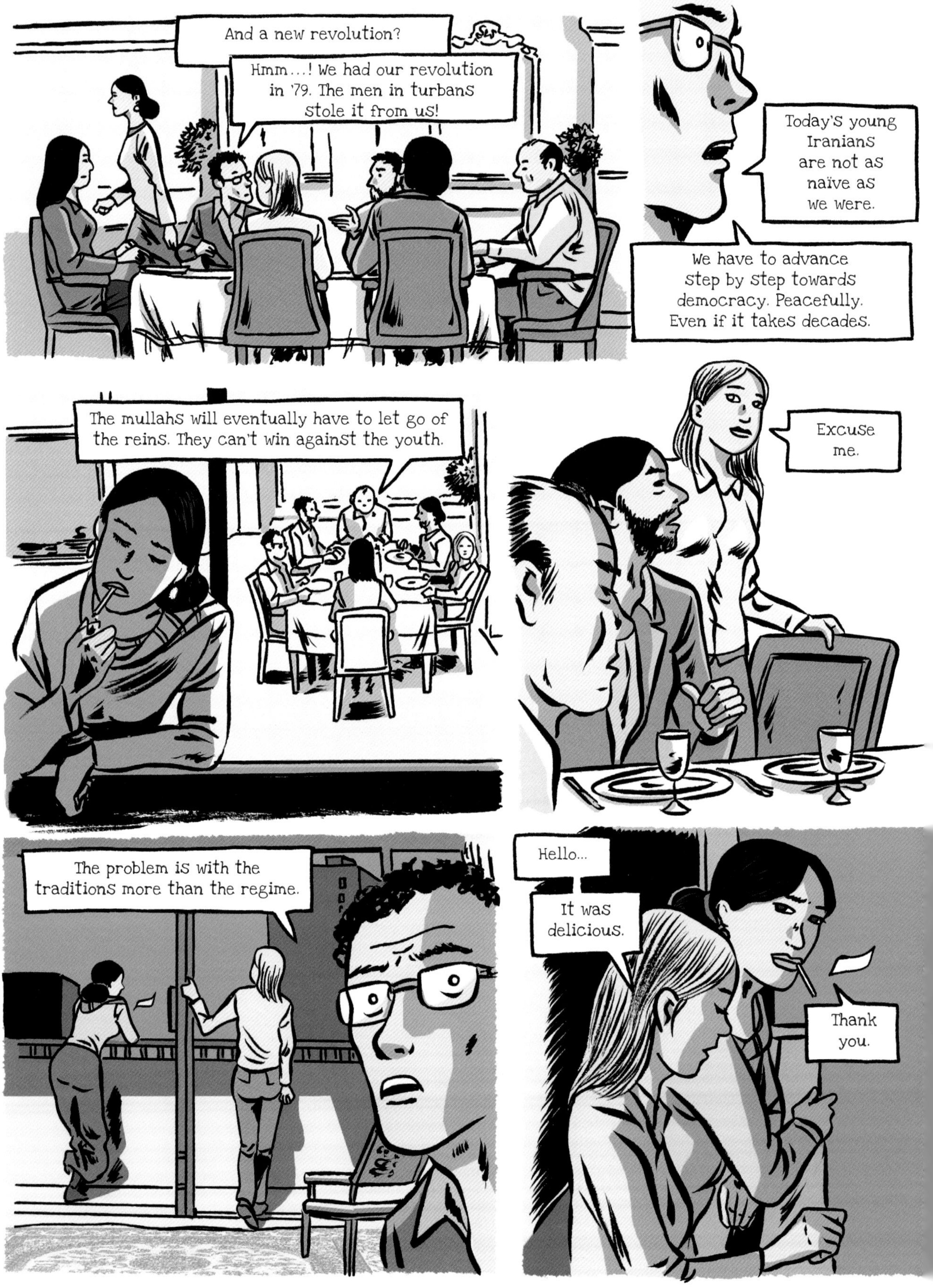
And a new revolution?
Hmm...! We had our revolution in '79. The men in turbans stole it from us!
Today's young Iranians are not as naïve as we were.
We have to advance step by step towards democracy. Peacefully. Even if it takes decades.
The mullahs will eventually have to let go of the reins. They can't win against the youth.
Excuse me.
The problem is with the traditions more than the regime.
Hello...
It was delicious.
Thank you.

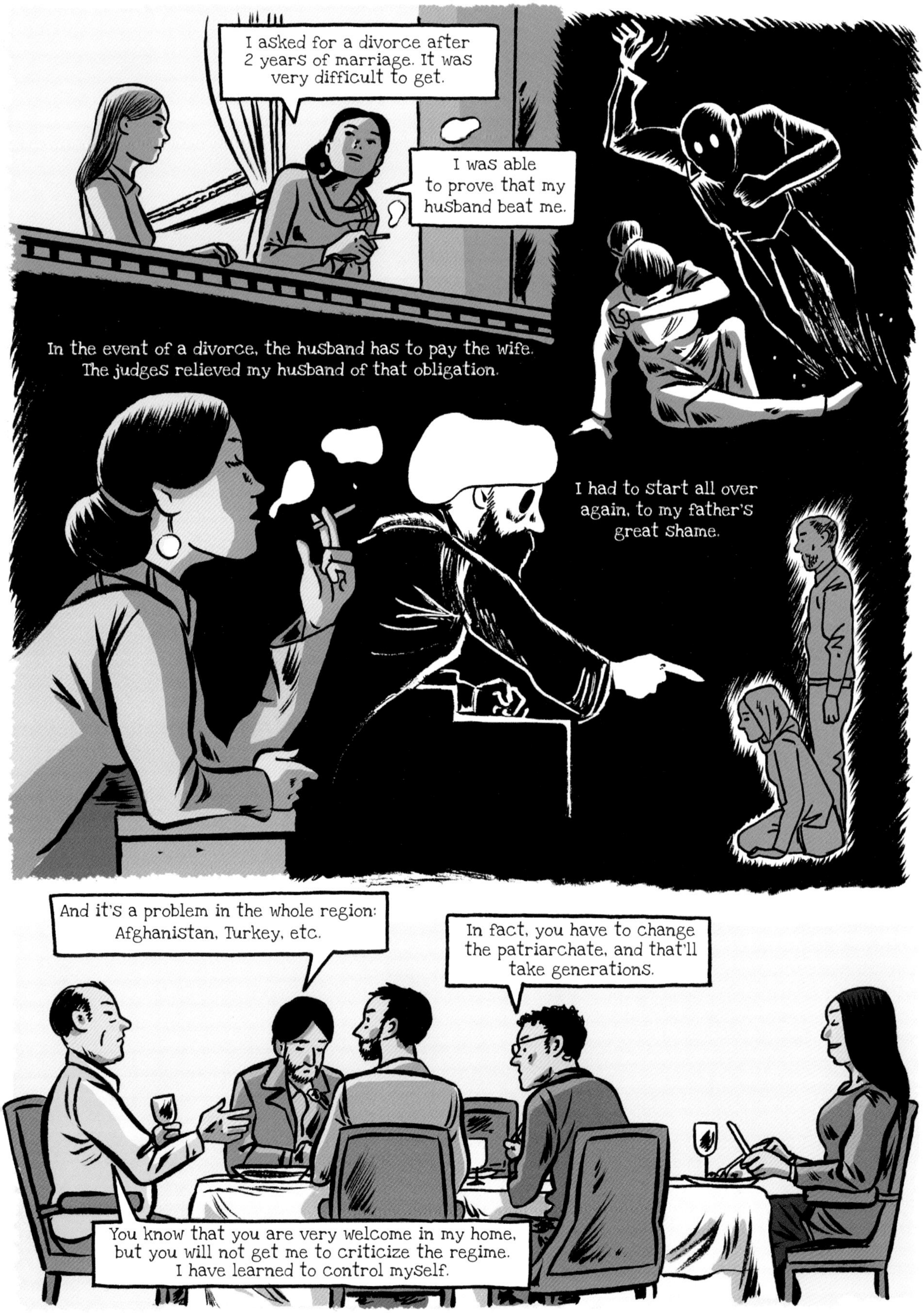
I asked for a divorce after 2 years of marriage. It was very difficult to get.
I was able to prove that my husband beat me.
In the event of a divorce, the husband has to pay the wife. The judges relieved my husband of that obligation.
I had to start all over again, to my father's great shame.
And it's a problem in the whole region: Afghanistan, Turkey, etc.
In fact, you have to change the patriarchate, and that'll take generations.
You know that you are very welcome in my home, but you will not get me to criticize the regime. I have learned to control myself.

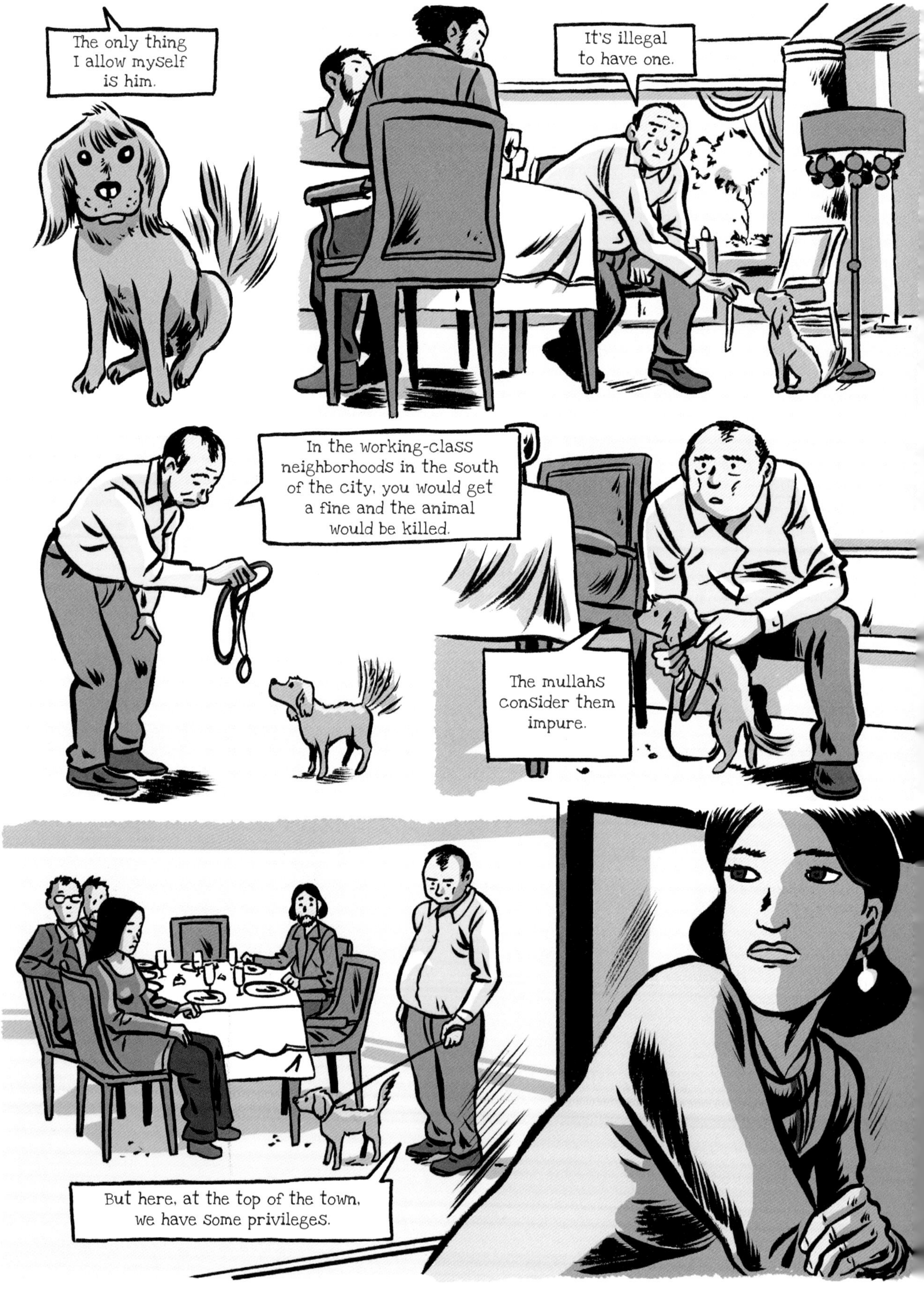
The only thing I allow myself is him.
It's illegal to have one.
In the working-class neighborhoods in the south of the city, you would get a fine and the animal would be killed.
The mullahs consider them impure.
But here, at the top of the town, we have some privileges.

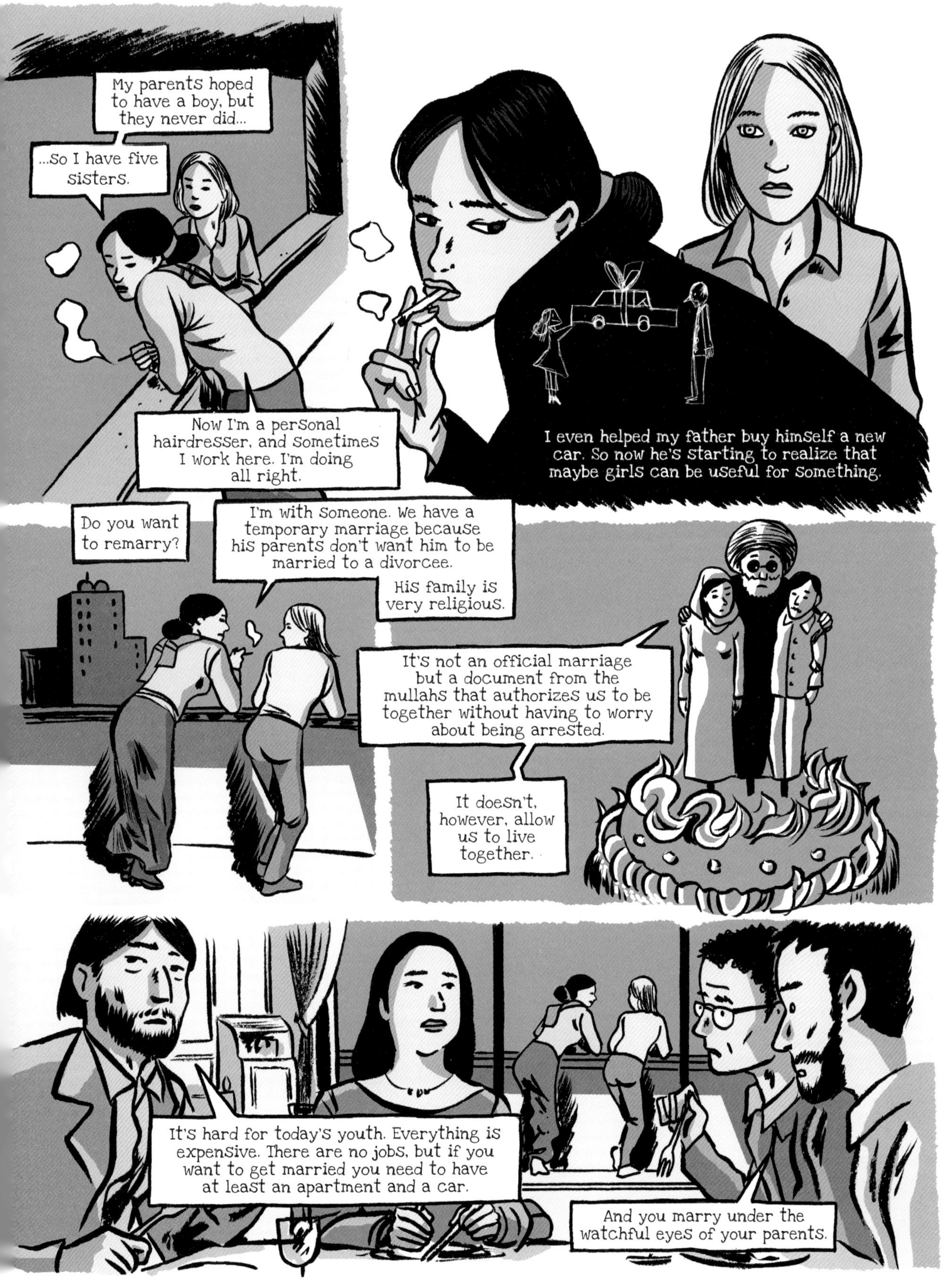

My parents hoped to have a boy, but they never did...
...So I have five sisters.
Now I'm a personal hairdresser, and sometimes I work here. I'm doing all right.
I even helped my father buy himself a new car. So now he's starting to realize that maybe girls can be useful for something.
Do you want to remarry?
I'm with someone. We have a temporary marriage because his parents don't want him to be married to a divorcee.
His family is very religious.
It's not an official marriage but a document from the mullahs that authorizes us to be together without having to worry about being arrested.
It doesn't, however, allow us to live together.
It's hard for today's youth. Everything is expensive. There are no jobs, but if you want to get married you need to have at least an apartment and a car.
And you marry under the watchful eyes of your parents.

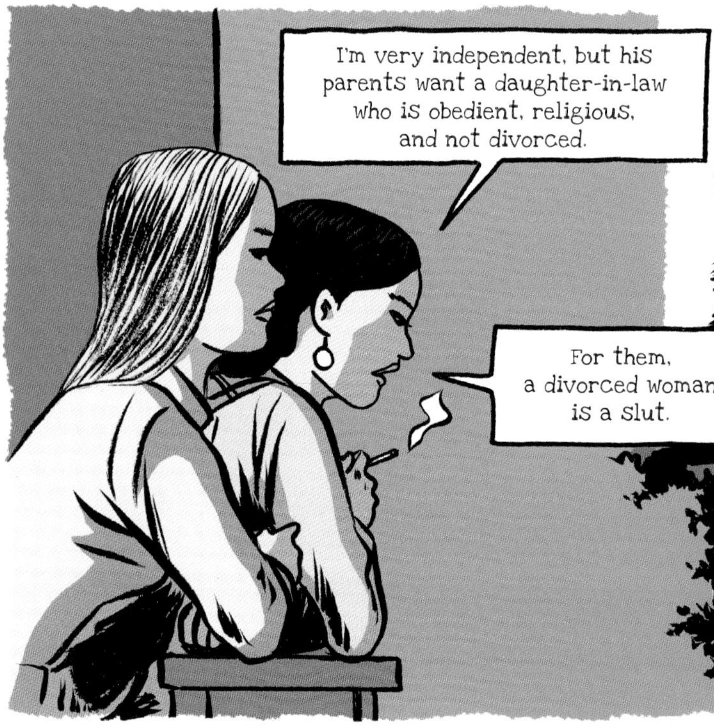
I'm very independent, but his parents want a daughter-in-law who is obedient, religious, and not divorced.
For them, a divorced woman is a slut.

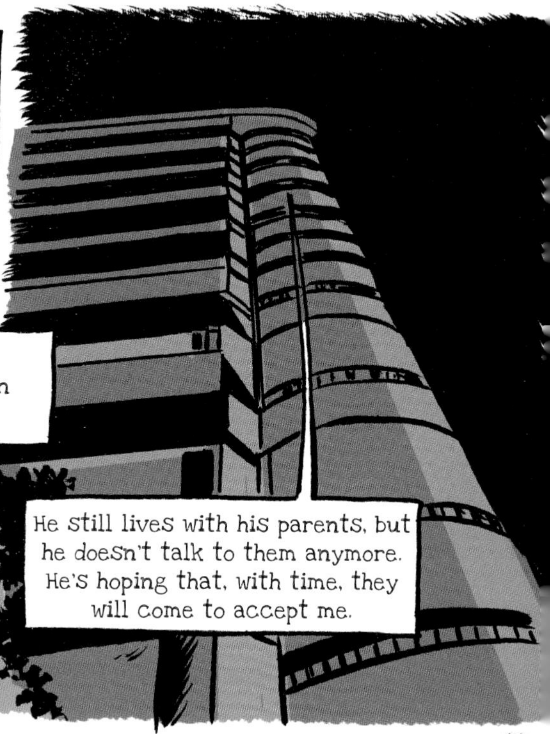
He still lives with his parents, but he doesn't talk to them anymore. He's hoping that, with time, they will come to accept me.

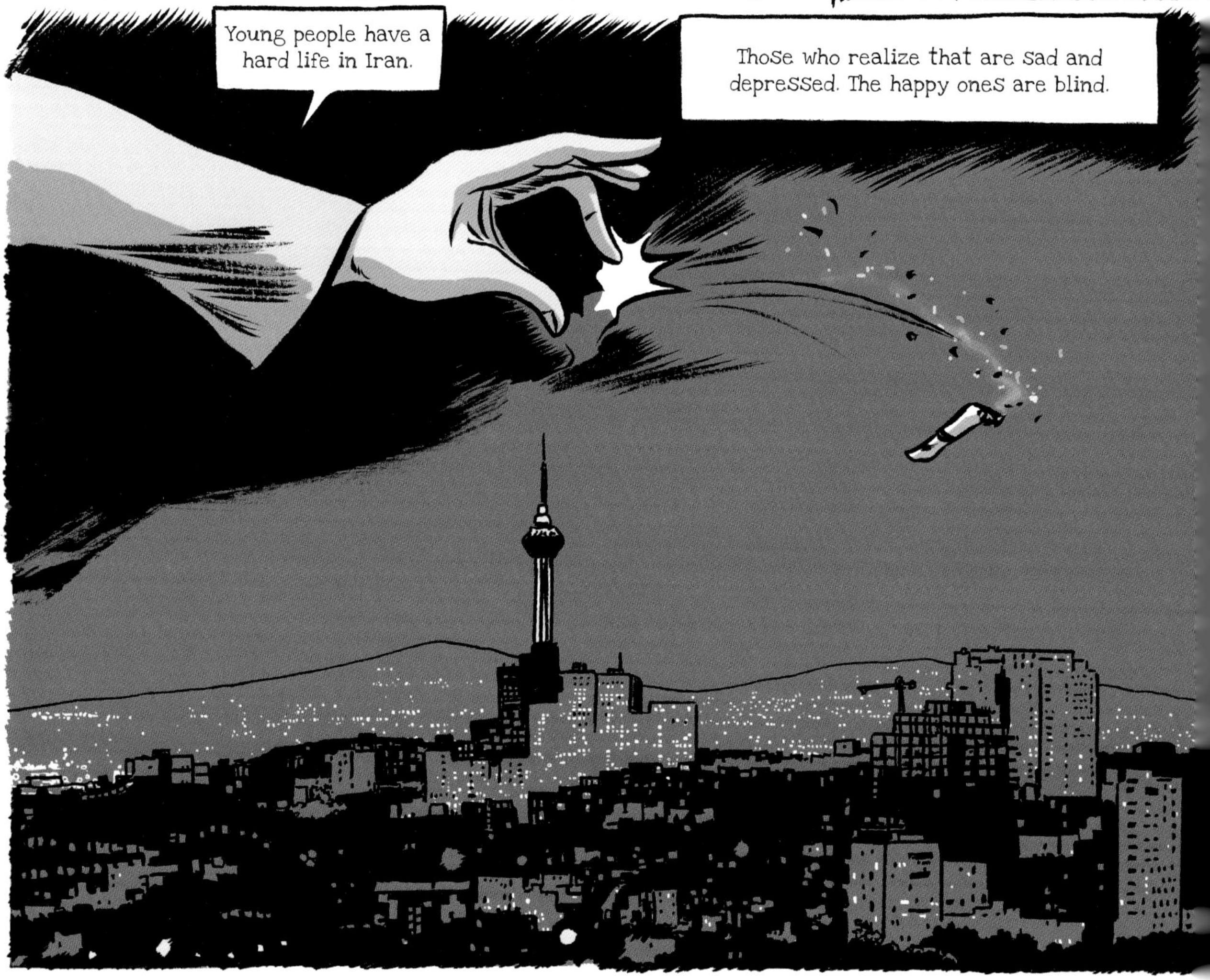
Young people have a hard life in Iran.
Those who realize that are sad and depressed. The happy ones are blind.

We left the country...

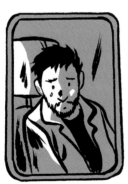 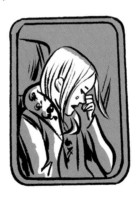 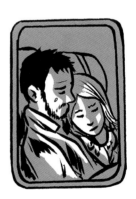

The pressure dropped.

To the Iranians who agreed to tell us their stories, and to those who didn't dare.
To all the Iranians: It's an honor to have met you.

Library of Congress Cataloging-in-Publication Data

Names: Deuxard, Jane, author. | Deloupy, 1968– illustrator. | Hahnenberger,
    Ivanka, translator.
Title: Iranian love stories / script, Jane Deuxard ; art, Deloupy ; translated
    by Ivanka Hahnenberger.
Other titles: Love story à l'iranienne. English
Description: University Park, Pennsylvania : Graphic Mundi, [2021] |
    "Originally published in French under the following title: Love Story à
    l'iranienne by Jane Deuxard and Deloupy, © Editions Delcourt—2016."
Summary: "A series of vignettes, in graphic novel format, that explore the
    lives of ten young Iranian men and women from diverse backgrounds"—
    Provided by publisher.
Identifiers: LCCN 2021018934 | ISBN 9781637790045 (hardback)
Subjects: LCSH: Young adults—Iran—Comic books, strips, etc. | Man-
    woman relationships—Iran—Comic books, strips, etc. | Civil rights—
    Iran—Comic books, strips, etc. | Iran—Social life and customs—21st cen-
    tury—Comic books, strips, etc. | Iran—History—Election protests,
    2009—Comic books, strips, etc. | LCGFT: Graphic novels.
Classification: LCC DS318.82 .D4813 2021 | DDC 955.06/1092542—dc23
LC record available at https://lccn.loc.gov/2021018934

Copyright © 2021 The Pennsylvania State University
All rights reserved
Printed in Lithuania
Published by The Pennsylvania State University Press,
University Park, PA 16802-1003

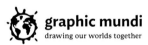

Graphic Mundi is an imprint of The Pennsylvania State University Press.

Translated by Ivanka Hahnenberger

Originally published in French under the following title:
Love Story à l'iranienne by Jane Deuxard and Deloupy
© Editions Delcourt – 2016

The Pennsylvania State University Press is a member of the Association of
University Presses.

It is the policy of The Pennsylvania State University Press to use acid-free
paper. Publications on uncoated stock satisfy the minimum requirements
of American National Standard for Information Sciences—Permanence of
Paper for Printed Library Material, ANSI Z39.48–1992.